Pregnancy
Sucks

Pregnancy Sucks

What to Do
When Your **Miracle**
Makes You **Miserable**

Joanne Kimes with
Sanford A. Tisherman, M.D.

Adams Media
Avon, Massachusetts

Published by
Adams Media, an F+W Publications Company
57 Littlefield Street, Avon MA 02322 U.S.A.
www.adamsmedia.com

ISBN: 1-58062-934-2

Printed in the Untied States of America

J I H G F E D C

Library of Congress Cataloging-in-Publication Data
Kimes, Joanne.
Pregnancy sucks / Joanne Kimes with Sanford A. Tisherman.
p.   cm.
ISBN 1-58062-934-2
1. Pregnancy—Popular works. 2. Childbirth—Popular works.
[DNLM: 1. Pregnancy—Popular Works. 2. Delivery, Obstetric—
Popular Works. 3. Puerperium—Popular Works. WQ 150 K49p 2003]
I. Tisherman, Sanford A. II. Title.

RG525.K499 2003
618.2—dc21
2003004459

This publication is designed to provide accurate and authoritative information with regard to the subject matter covered. It is sold with the understanding that the publisher is not engaged in rendering legal, accounting, or other professional advice. If legal advice or other expert assistance is required, the services of a competent professional person should be sought.
　　　　　—From a *Declaration of Principles* jointly adopted by a Committee
of the American Bar Association and a Committee of Publishers and Associations

This publication is designed to provide accurate and authoritative information with regard to the subject matter covered. It is sold with the understanding that the publisher is not engaged in rendering professional medical advice. If assistance is required, the services of a competent professional person should be sought.

Many of the designations used by manufacturers and sellers to distinguish their products are claimed as trademarks. Where those designations appear in this book and Adams Media was aware of a trademark claim, the designations have been printed with initial capital letters.

Cover photo by Andreas Pollok/Getty Images.

This book is available at quantity discounts for bulk purchases.
For information, call 1-800-872-5627.

*I dedicate this book, and my life,
to my precious daughter Emily.
I love you more than cookie dough.*

Contents

Chapter Eleven: Home, Bittersweet Home . . . 211

Acknowledgments

eing a busy stay-at-home mom, I found it an enormous challenge to write a book (it's hard enough just finding the time to even read one). But, thanks to some incredible people, the task was completed and a dream was fulfilled. Because of this, I want to take a moment to thank them.

First and foremost, thank you to my wonderful husband, Jeff. There would never have even been a book without your overwhelming love, incredible support, and fertile reproductive system.

To my editor, Kate Epstein, I'm forever grateful that you pulled my proposal out from your towering slush pile, and took a chance with it and me. This book is much better thanks to your creative ideas.

To Dr. Sandy Tisherman. I'm so glad that you agreed to share your medical advice and pregnancy secrets. You're an amazing doctor and approve so many more medications than I was allowed, that I almost wish that I were pregnant again. Almost.

And thanks to my mom for taking my daughter out every Wednesday so that I could work, even when she was cranky (my daughter, not my mom). Without your help, I'd still be on the table of contents.

And thanks to my dad, for telling me as a child that I had talent to write. It makes it easier to believe in yourself when someone you love believes in you first.

I'm also indebted to Nurse Sharron, my family, friends, and even complete strangers, who generously contributed their advice and pregnancy suckage stories for all to share and enjoy.

And finally, a big thanks to Po, my daughter's favorite Teletubbie, for keeping her entertained while Mommy had a deadline.

Introduction

A Book Is Born

*I*f there's one thing I've known for sure about myself, it's that I've wanted kids. My biological clock started ticking during my first menstrual cramp, and it ticked loud and clear. It was like carrying Big Ben around in my uterus. But, as much as I knew that I wanted children, I wasn't as sure that I wanted to be pregnant. Nine months of bloating and back-aches and hemorrhoids, oh my! And then, after enduring these long agonizing months, I'd have to push out a kid the size of a toaster through an opening the size of a tampon. What a horrible design flaw. Can't we learn anything from the marsupial?

But pregnancy was never much of an issue for me until I met an incredible man and we fell in love. (I figured that God was making it up to me for having me need braces.) We got married and decided to be good little procreators and have a baby. Who knows, I figured, maybe I'd be wrong. Maybe I'd go through my nine months without even one complaint. Maybe I'd be like one of those pregnant supermodels who, in their ninth month, look like I do after eating Thanksgiving dinner.

But unfortunately, it wasn't to be. As my pregnancy progressed, all my dreaded fears came true . . . and then some. Sure, I knew to expect morning sickness and backaches, but why didn't anyone tell me about Braxton Hicks? Why wasn't I warned about a third nipple? Was there a secret pact amongst mothers to never tell the truth to us childless women for fear they'd be alone in their misery?

Tormented and confused, I went to the local bookstore and read everything I could about pregnancy. But I discovered that none of the books ever went far enough in telling me the true horrors of reproduction. What the books described as a mild discomfort, I would describe as unthinkable agony. I needed help. I needed guidance. I needed to reverse time and consider adoption.

I asked for help from friends of mine who had kids, and time and time again I'd hear the same thing: that being pregnant was the best time of their lives. I don't know why I asked these fools anyway. They thought the same was true about high school. They tried to put me at ease by saying that once I had my child, it would all be worth it. Let me tell you, there were times so difficult I thought the only way this would all be worth it is if my kid came out holding a winning lottery ticket.

There was obviously something very wrong with me. For some reason, my body was having an adverse reaction to pregnancy. Was I the only woman who felt like this? Were there any others out there drowning in a sea of sciatica? Anyone else who felt like less of a woman just because she wished that she were born a man?

Sure, there are some women who do love being pregnant. They experience no morning sickness or any other discomfort during their nine months. They have bodies that were born to breed. But if you're one of the women who are feeling the same way that I did, pregnant and hating it, then this book is for you. I want to share my experiences with you to show you that you're not alone. I want to pass on any advice I have in hopes of making your nine months more bearable. I want to tell you that there is nothing to be ashamed of. The truth is, *pregnancy can suck!*

I hope that by reading this book, you'll learn a few things about what to do if you're having a rough time. And maybe, by seeing all the things that *can* go wrong, by comparison you may not think that your pregnancy experience sucks as much as you thought it did. I hope that by the end of these nine months, your pregnancy can teach you something about yourself, for I know that it taught me one very valuable lesson: That my daughter will definitely be an only child.

Chapter One

The First Month

Congratulations, you did it! You got knocked up! I don't know about you, but the whole process of conception was quite a bit more than I had expected. I ignorantly thought that if you had unprotected sex, you'd conceive. I didn't know you needed the accuracy of a moon launch to make a sperm make contact with an egg.

To begin with, I was at the advanced age of thirty-five when I ventured down the path of procreation. This meant that my window of opportunity to conceive had shrunk from the size of a garage door to that of a peephole. If my husband and I stayed to watch the end credits of a movie, we could blow it until the next month.

At first I tried the basal thermometer method. That's the one where you *must* take your temperature every morning before you get out of bed. (I can't tell you how many times I remembered that while I was sitting on the toilet each morning.)

Next, I looked into the vaginal discharge method. Although it's been used throughout the ages, I found the process of searching myself for "egg white" rather gross. So, I turned to medical science. I bought an ovulation predictor kit, peed on a stick, and had sex three nights in a row as instructed. A couple of weeks later I took a pregnancy test and saw the two lines that I had been praying for! I was pregnant! I was the happiest that I'd ever been. Little did I know that my pregnancy experience was at its peak.

For days, I was in a constant state of euphoria. I was looking forward to my turn as a proud mama-to-be. I was going to look like those beautiful pregnant women on book covers and glide through these next nine months with a soft focus lens and a constant smile. Sure, I was prepared to eat a cracker once in a while, and knew that there might be an ache or pain along the way, but how bad could it really be?

But every month seemed to bring an unexpected bombardment of pregnancy ailments. And it seemed that as soon as one misery dissipated, another one took its place. I've jotted down the ailments that I had (and some others that I didn't but threw in for good measure), and when I experienced them. Your trip down your own road of gestation may be different than mine, filled with its own unique twists and turns. You may get some ailments earlier than I did, some later on, or I hope, not at all. But, in general, each month will bring on its own unique roadblock that you'll have to plow through. I'll explain each one to you in detail and offer my advice on how to ease the distress that going forth and multiplying can bring.

Choosing an O.B.

The first thing that you'll want to do after you pass your pregnancy test is look for an obstetrician. Not only do you want him (or her, but I'm going to use "him" since mine was a "him") to confirm the results of your pregnancy test, you're going to want to start your prenatal care as soon as possible.

I put a lot of research into choosing my obstetrician. I asked for recommendations. I went over references. Then, after realizing how expensive it would be otherwise, I chose the doctor covered by my insurance plan. I was skeptical at first. I didn't know anything about him or anyone who went to him. But I figured I'd at least give him a try. If I didn't like him, we'd shell out the big bucks and later push our child into going to a community college.

While waiting for my first visit, the background check began. I asked several of his other patients waiting with me, and they all raved about the doctor, saying that he was a wonderful man. A couple of the women were even going back to him for their second and third babies! Repeat customers, now that's high praise.

When I finally met my doctor I liked him right away. He was knowledgeable, personable, and had an air of confidence that made me feel like everything was going to be okay in his hands. And what a pair of hands they were. For some reason they were incredibly huge and puffy. Each finger was like a cooked Ball Park Frank. If anyone could safely catch my newborn as it fell from my uterus into the world, it would be him.

I hope you'll be fortunate enough to have a choice in picking an obstetrician. You may even be deciding between several of them. If that's the case, let me offer some suggestions on how to choose one. I'm assuming that they'll be board certified and have good references from friends or family. Also, that they have privileges at the hospital where you wish to deliver, and agree to any specific birth plan that you may have in mind. But, assuming all is equal, here are a few suggestions that may put one over the top and help you decide which one to pick:

1. Which doctor's office is closer? You'll be going to your doctor often. You'll probably have a checkup every four weeks for the first six months, then one every other week until the last month, when you will go every week. And in between your checkups you'll need blood workups and glucose tests and genetic evaluations, and so on. If you lease your car, a doctor who is far away could put you over your mileage limit.

2. Does he have an in-house ultrasound machine? My O.B. didn't have an ultrasound machine available at his office, but many do. Whenever I needed to have an ultrasound, I had to make another appointment somewhere else.

3. What's your O.B.'s vacation schedule? Obstetricians have a demanding life. They treat patients during office hours, and can also be up all night delivering babies. This hectic workload can make for a doctor who desperately needs a vacation. But you don't want his vacation to be anywhere near your due date.

4. How far do some of his patients travel to see him? I know this doctor in Los Angeles who has patients from as far away as San Diego. You gotta think that if a patient is willing to drive up to two hours for an office visit, he must be damn good.

5. What is his list of acceptable medications? Not all O.B.s agree when it comes to taking medications. Some dissuade you from taking any medications at all while others disperse them freely. My personal advice is to choose the doctor who allows for the most kinds of medications. You don't have to take them if you don't want to, but they're there if you do.

6. What magazines does he subscribe to? You'll no

doubt be spending a great deal of time in the waiting room. I would try to make my appointments either the first one of the day or the first after lunch so the wait would be less, but it didn't always help. I still had to wait. But my doctor had fantastic magazines that made the waiting time easier.

7. Does he practice in a group or as an individual? If he's in a group, you may not be seeing him at every visit but rather may alternate with other partners in the group. Also, you'll want to find out if he'll be the one who delivers your baby instead of another doctor whom you may not be as comfortable with.

As the months went on, I found myself developing a slight crush on my doctor. I hear this is pretty common. Maybe it's because your doctor will care about your unborn child as much as you will. Maybe it's because of all the support he'll give you during this emotional time. Or maybe it's because he takes the time to read all the pregnancy books that you can't get your own husband to look at. No matter the reason, don't be surprised if you put on your sexiest muumuu before each appointment.

The No-No List

I guess it's all a matter of give-and-take. Now that you've been given one of the greatest gifts of life, some of the greatest pleasures are going to be taken away. I knew about the biggies I'd have to abstain from once I conceived, but there were many more that I was unaware of. Here is a partial list of pregnancy no-no's you too should adhere to:

- Alcohol
- Cigarettes

- Caffeine (Some doctors believe a small amount is okay.)
- Excess chocolate (it has caffeine)
- Heating pads turned on high
- Drugs (except those prescribed by your doctor)
- Soft cheeses like goat and Brie (if you can cut it with a butter knife, you should probably steer clear)
- Chemical hair dyes (most all doctors agree that vegetable dyes and hennas are best during pregnant)
- Diet drinks (or anything that contains an artificial sweetener)
- Hot showers (very hot temperatures can cause birth defects)
- Hot tubs (same reason as hot showers)
- Electric blankets (same reason as hot tubs and showers)
- Microwaves (don't stand in front of them)
- Changing the litter box (you could get toxoplasmosis)
- Sushi (you could get parasites)
- Aerobic class (during the first trimester if you're not used to them)
- Bikini waxing (just for the first trimester because of the risk of an infected ingrown hair)
- Air travel (during the last eight to ten weeks of pregnancy)
- Insecticides
- X-rays (unless essential and approved by your O.B.)
- Strong chemical fumes (oven cleaner, gasoline, etc.)

I say this is a partial list because by the time this book comes out they may have come up with another major no-no that's destined to cause your belly buddy some harm.

My mom never understood it when I passed up coffee at dinner or skipped the chocolate cake. She said that people are too educated these days. In her day she could eat or drink or smoke anything she wanted and everything turned out just fine. It was much better back then. I ranted and raved that in her day there were also many more underweight and premature babies, as well as babies with birth defects, immature lungs and even worse, babies who were stillborn. She didn't say anymore about it . . . ever.

It's very frustrating that there is so much you have to deny yourself when you're pregnant. It would be much easier to enjoy yourself in your condition if there were a different kind of list of no-no's to adhere to. I'd like to propose the following things that one must also abstain from when with child:

1. Doing dishes
2. Running errands
3. Using a computer
4. Pretreating laundry
5. Killing household insects
6. Driving people to the airport
7. Enduring bad hair days
8. Cleaning out a raw chicken
9. Waiting in line
10. Being on hold
11. Paying full price
12. Folding fitted sheets

If you're one of the "they" people—"they" say you have to do this, and "they" say you have to do that—I'd like for you to consider the above list. It would make enduring pregnancy so much more enjoyable. Thank you for your time.

Sore Boobs

One of the first symptoms of pregnancy that you'll no doubt experience will be sore breasts. Every pregnant woman I know had this symptom. It's just like the tender, achy feeling that you experienced when you had your periods, only super-sized.

Having sore boobs can be quite frustrating for those desperately trying to conceive. You struggle to calculate your fertile time, wait those endless two weeks to see if you've hit the jackpot, then suddenly, as you near the end of your cycle, your boobs begin to ache. Are they sore because you're pregnant, or are they sore because they always are before your period?

In general, most early pregnancy symptoms are the same ones as menstrual symptoms so it's difficult to tell which you're experiencing. Are you yelling because you're having a mood swing or is it just PMS? Are you late because you conceived, or because you're stressed out from trying? This is a cruel joke Mother Nature plays on her innocent little children.

I'm not sure why the boobs even need to get involved at this point of the pregnancy game. They don't really play into the whole baby picture until after the kid is born, and then it's suppertime! If you ask me, those glands are a little too ambitious, definitely a type A personality.

You may find that the most frustrating thing of all about sore boobs is that it makes tummy sleeping quite difficult. I don't know about you, but for me there's no other position quite as comfy. But, with those swollen mammaries in the way, it's impossible to lie on your stomach without aches and pains. And to make matters even more infuriating, the breast tenderness starts to go away around the fourth month of pregnancy, which is the same time that your belly will get too big to sleep on!

> **"** My breasts ached so bad that I went to the beach
> and dug a hole in the sand so I could lie down
> without pain. It felt too good, because I fell asleep
> and woke up three hours later with a sunburn that
> hurt far worse than my breasts ever did. **"**
> —Julie

Just like premenstrual breast tenderness, there's not much to do about it. I only have a pittance of advice to give:

1. Don't wear an underwire bra.
2. If you must wear one, buy one that's one size bigger than you need. This way there's room for your breasts to roam free, and the wire that's there to lift and support won't smush and contort.
3. Avoid standing in wind tunnels, or living in Chicago. A strong gust can really make those puppies ache.

The pain in your breasts should ease by about the third or fourth month. And by that time they'll amaze you, if you were small breasted to begin with. For your tiny boobs will grow like giant water balloons. You'll finally have those large firm breasts that you've always dreamt of. But, if you were fairly large breasted to begin with like me, that dream will become a nightmare.

I was one of those girls who started developing early and I always felt uncomfortable with my ample size. Besides, my personality is more spunky than voluptuous. I'm like a breast-transsexual—a small-breasted personality trapped in a full-figured woman. So, when my pregnancy boobs started to grow in, I became scared of them. I looked at myself in the mirror and saw the chest of my bosomy Aunt Florence.

I remember once as a child going to her house and seeing her change into a bathing suit. When I saw those overgrown protrusions staring down at me, I ran far and I ran fast. But now that they were on me, there was no place to run.

I can't suggest anything that will deflate your pregnancy breasts, so get used to them. They come in quite handy to rest a dinner plate on when you're at a buffet. They'll also keep you safe from drowning. I do recommend that you treat these titties with care. From my own personal experience, I strongly suggest that you invest in a good support bra. I had good bras to begin with, but when my pregnancy boobs arrived, I knew I needed to bring in the heavy artillery. I bought several bras throughout my pregnancy to keep up with the expansion, and they all were well constructed. These things strapped my breasts in place like a house bolted to its foundation.

I also suggest that you wear your bra from the moment you conceive until the day you stop breastfeeding—morning, noon, *and* night. Not to brag, but my breasts don't look that much worse for the wear (not that they were all that great to begin with), and I really think it's because of all the support I gave those girls during those long and strenuous months.

Morning, Noon, and Night Sickness

I had been floating on a cloud for a week after I passed my pregnancy test. There was a smile on my face not even rush hour traffic could wipe away. But then, it happened. I was run over by a truck. Not an actual truck, mind you, but it felt as if it had been. It hit me without warning and it hit me hard. I was struck with morning sickness.

I know that for some incredibly lucky people, probably the same ones who can eat anything they want without getting fat, morning sickness doesn't strike at all. Or at the least, it can be cured by eating a cracker. For me, it was so powerful, that, at times, it made me wish that I'd never gotten pregnant. I know that sounds harsh, but being pregnant can induce a state of temporary insanity.

Morning sickness is like waking up every day for three months with a terrible flu. It usually begins in the fifth or sixth week of pregnancy and lingers until about the fourteenth. It doesn't creep up on you but comes on with a vengeance. It drains you of your spirit and takes away your ability to care about anything. The fridge is broken? Who cares, you're nauseated. The dog's fur just fell off? Not your problem. You're weak. I can't believe that some mothers-to-be have to endure this kind of misery. Morning sickness gave me a whole new respect for womankind, and made me swear that I'd never raise my voice to my mother again.

Whoever named it morning sickness was terribly mistaken. The name implies that you only feel bad when the day begins. It gives you false hope that, as the day goes on, you'll start to feel better. But then you don't. At least I didn't. I suffered the entire day. I suggest that the name be changed to "morning-noon-and-night sickness." Truth be told, there was one point in each day that I wasn't in misery. For ten beautiful minutes each morning before I got out of bed, I felt no pain. I would lie there and remember what it felt like to be a human being.

No one knows the cause of morning sickness. One theory I heard is that morning sickness is the result of your body trying to rid itself of the infection you call your baby. It sees your offspring as a foreign matter that must be destroyed. Another theory is that morning sickness is caused by the increased level of progesterone in your system that keeps the baby alive. In fact, if you have severe morning sickness, the old wives say that you'll have a girl. You'll find that these wives have a lot to say during your pregnancy.

But even if no one can agree on the cause, they all agree on one thing. There is no cure. Believe me, if there were, I would have found it. I searched high and low. I asked doctors and surfed the Internet. I couldn't believe there was no pill to cure my ill. It's barbaric. There should be a team of researchers working around the clock. There should be a clinic in every city across the nation devoted to find a cure. There should be a yearly telethon with a poster child of a green bloated woman clutching hard on to a toilet bowl.

Unlike any other illness, don't expect morning sickness to get you a lot of sympathy—except from other women who have gone through it themselves. Your friends and family will be too excited that you're pregnant to really pity you the way you deserve. I remember lying facedown on my office floor, and whenever someone came in, they would just look at me and smile. There was no "Can I get you anything?" or "Why don't you go home?" There was just a damn smile. Maybe if morning sickness came with the physical symptoms it deserves—like convulsions or dismemberment—it would get the proper recognition.

So, let's get down to the burning question: What can you do to feel better? When I had morning sickness, I asked every pregnant woman I saw if she had any advice. I'd stop them in the produce section. I'd corner them in elevators. I'd hope beyond hope that they would utter some words of wisdom that would get me through this terrible time. I found many of these women to be very knowledgeable. I got several different suggestions, which I'll pass along to you.

1. Sea bands. They're soft wristbands you can get at a drug store that you wear tightly on each wrist. They were originally created to ease the nausea caused by motion sickness. They have a hard plastic ball on the inside of them that presses against your wrist. This is a pressure point in acupuncture that helps with nausea.

2. Lemon wedges. The theory behind this is that if you're nauseated, take a bite of a slice of lemon. Your brain can't react to both the nausea and the bitter taste of the lemon at the same time, and since the taste of the lemon is stronger, it wins out. You may feel as though you've eroded the enamel off your teeth, but at least you won't feel sick.

3. Ginger. Supposedly, it's a natural nausea reliever. You can try crystallized ginger, ginger tea, or better yet, just gnaw on a chunk of raw ginger root.

4. Eat protein with carbohydrates. Many women told me that they felt much better after eating cheese and crackers, a tuna fish sandwich (if you can tolerate the smell), or any combination of protein and carbohydrates together.

5. Black licorice. I met a woman at a barbecue who swore by black licorice. I ate several pieces, but the only thing it helped me cure was my sweet tooth.

6. Raspberry tea. Dafna, my friend who is a midwife, told me about this. I always gave it more clout because of that. Although it didn't cure my morning sickness, I rather liked the taste and still drink it to this day.

I gave all of these suggestions a try and, although some may have eased the distress somewhat, nothing took it away completely. So, I turned to my doctor. Luckily, he was a firm believer in over-the-counter medication. My doctor's remedies did help to soften the green around my gills, so I'll tell you what he said. Be sure to ask your doctor if these medicines are okay, and if they are, ask him what dosage you need to take. It may be different than the dosage on the package. He may also have some other tricks up his sleeve, and if he does, I suggest that you try them all.

1. **Benadryl.** It's an antihistamine that will make you drowsy. Not only will this calm you down, but it might also calm down your tummy.
2. **Emetrol.** It's like cola without the bubbles and is specifically marketed to help relieve nausea. You can buy this over the counter at most drug stores.
3. **Dramamine.** This is medicine used to alleviate sea sickness.
4. **Vitamin B$_6$.** If you are having trouble keeping your prenatal vitamins down, your doctor might prescribe some that have extra vitamin B$_6$ as this has been proved to quell that queasiness.
5. **Unisom.** Yes, I know it's marketed as a sleep aid, and indeed it may make you drowsy, but it may also make you feel better. If your doctor allows, take half a tablet with 50 milligrams B$_6$.

I came up with a few suggestions of my own, too. First of all, take caution when it comes to your prenatal vitamin. Those pills are so strong they can cause nausea all by themselves. Don't take it all at one time. I suggest half in the morning and half at night. If that's still too strong, break it into thirds, or fourths, or twelfths—or just put it on a stick and lick it throughout the day. During the worst of my morning sickness, I skipped my prenatal altogether, and took my everyday vitamin. Yes, I told my doctor first. I know you're thinking I'm a horrible mother depriving my helpless embryo of its nourishment, but how much riboflavin does a ten-cell organism need? Besides, my doctor told me that the embryo took all the nutrients it needed from me, so those pills were actually to keep *me* healthy. I don't know about you, but I survived an entire college semester on Doritos and cookie dough. I was going to be just fine. If you find that your prenatal vitamins are making your stomach uneasy, ask your doctor if you can skip them as well. As long as you take a one-milligram tablet of folic acid daily, he may not have a problem with it. You can also try switching the brand of your prenatal vitamin. Not all prenatal vitamins are created equal.

Also, NEVER take your prenatal vitamin on an empty stomach. It will make you sick so fast your head will spin (or at least it'll spin after you've puked). It's important always to keep something in your stomach, anyway. You should put some crackers by your bed and have a couple before you even get up in the morning. I know you don't feel the least bit hungry, but do it. I ate a bunch of little meals throughout the day. About forty-five to be truthful. Don't force yourself to eat something that might make you sick, but find something you can tolerate and stick with it. Comfort foods usually work well. I found myself drinking a lot of Slurpees, something I hadn't had since I owned a "Close and Play."

Also, be extra careful brushing your back teeth. I don't know why it happens, but all of a sudden putting a toothbrush in the back of your mouth is going to make you throw up. I suspect that there's some type of gag reflex that starts up in the first stages of pregnancy. You can be feeling perfectly fine and then, out of nowhere, BLECH! So just focus on the front teeth and avoid talking throughout the day. This shouldn't be much of a problem since your sallow complexion will be a tip-off to those around you that you're not in the mood for stimulating conversation.

I hope that these suggestions will make you feel better. But even if they don't, keep in mind things could be worse. You could have been born an elephant. Their gestation period is about two and a half times as long as ours, which means that they spend about eight months in morning sickness misery. In my lowest moments, I found this to be a comfort.

Gas!

From almost the moment you conceive, your body does an amazing thing. Your digestive system slows down, allowing it time to squeeze out every nutrient it can from your food. This process, albeit a miraculous design of nature, makes you toot. They say there's a glow about a pregnant woman. The glow is undoubtedly the stress she's enduring trying not to cut one right in front of you.

You can try eliminating certain foods from your diet such as cabbage or beans. I didn't find that this made much of a difference. Even ice water played havoc on my innards. You can try eating small meals, avoiding tight waistbands, and sleeping with your head elevated. You can try strapping a monkey on your butt for all the good that'll do either. Or you can try taking some of my advice, such as the following.

> **"** Once, after a long meeting, I went to my office and let out the gas I'd been holding in for so long. Just then, the whole staff came in to surprise me with a 'congratulations on being pregnant' cake. I think they were as surprised as I was. **"**
>
> —Lisa

1. Request your own office.
2. Learn to say "Excuse me" in several different languages. This won't cure the gas, but you'll be improving your mind, which is always a good thing.
3. Practice squishing up your nose in disgust and looking around for the guilty party.
4. Suggest that your husband sleep on the couch. He'll no doubt be grateful for the permission.
5. Keep a window open at all times. Otherwise, you're not going to be able to stand being in the same room with yourself.

This kind of intestinal disturbance may have another side effect on you as well. It's an unusually hearty and consistent burp. It's not a burp exactly, more like a burp crossed with a hiccup. It's much louder than a burp and, like hiccups, comes on without any notice. And come on it does.

I would bur-cup so often it became second nature. After a while, I wasn't even aware of what I was doing. I would bur-cup in restaurants. Bur-cup in movie theaters. Bur-cup in meetings. Bur-cuping became as natural to me as breathing. It drove my husband insane. Once in a while he'd flash me a look like, "Can't you stop those stupid things already?" and I'd flash one right back that said, "Don't you dare criticize me when I'm feeling so miserable and you walk around everyday without vomiting or suffering any ill side effects at all from carrying around our child." Which brings me to another topic . . .

Resentment Toward Your Hubby

First of all, let me explain one thing. Whenever I refer to that special someone in your life, I'm going to call it "your husband." In your case, it may very well be a husband, but it might also be a boyfriend, a partner, a girlfriend, a lover, a dear friend, or maybe even a ferret. I don't know and I don't care. But, for simplicity sake, I'll just stick with "husband." Not only will it save me from doing a lot of extra typing (husband/boyfriend/girlfriend, etc.), but it will also be less confusing to the five remaining brain cells I have left after having a child (we'll get to that part later). So, with that understood, let us continue.

It's hard not to resent your husband when you're feeling like you're re-enacting the pea soup scene from *The Exorcist*, and he's walking around feeling "la-de-da" all day. I know it's irrational, but you may start to hate him. Okay, maybe "hate" is too strong a word. Let's just say that you'll loathe every cell in his body. It really is grossly unfair that the baby belongs to both of you, but the misery is yours and yours alone. And there's nothing, not one little thing that you can do to change that.

The only time my husband ever had any physical difficulty during the entire nine months of our pregnancy experience was during the third night of trying to conceive. He wasn't in the mood so he had to work at it, the poor dear.

But my husband is a good guy and did his best to try to help. Every day he would ask me what he could do for me, and every day I would answer the same way, "There's nothing, dear." But it didn't take long for my sickness to grow and my patience to fade, and my standard answer changed to, "You could carry the damn thing for just one day, you selfish bastard."

There are a couple of things you can do to lessen the resentment that you feel toward your spouse. First of all, insist that he do more things around the house. This won't lessen your resentment about carrying the child, but it will lessen your resentment about carrying the brunt of the household chores. If his constant pile of dirty socks is still at his bedside, ask him to put them away, or better yet, to do a load of whites. If you've always wanted shelves in the bathroom, now's the time to ask him to build them. Me, I wanted a new floor in the bathroom. Sure, tile work is hard but so is growing a child in your uterus.

Another way to relieve some of your resentment is to insist that your husband abstain from all the things that you must abstain from. No drink at the end of the day, or coffee after dinner and so on and so on and so on. You can even give him one of your prenatal vitamins (which he should take on an empty stomach) so he can experience the nausea along with you. What a bond you two will share! Not only will you feel less resentment toward him, but he'll also feel more compassion toward you. He'll put you up higher on your pedestal, which is exactly where a woman in your condition belongs.

I asked my husband to do this and he managed to give up most no-no's without any trouble. But the one no-no that he couldn't give up was smoking. He'd try to stop, but he just couldn't do it. After the baby was born, I insisted he quit. Not only did I love him and want him around for a long time, but, once I saw how hard childrearing was, I knew I didn't want to go at it alone. He tried patches and gum, and I tried yelling and guilt. But the thing that finally motivated him to stop was when I told him that I was going to start dating again. I figured that it could easily take a couple of years to find my next husband (a girl should be picky you know) and I didn't want to have such a lull in my matrimonial state. So he quit cold turkey. Imagine that.

Tests, Tests, and More Tests

Get out your number-two pencils ladies, there's going to be a test. Actually, there are going to be quite a lot of them. The entrance exam is already over. That was the pregnancy test, and I'm assuming that you aced it or you wouldn't be reading this book. But there's a college course load still to be done, so let's start cracking.

The first series of tests will take place during your first doctor's visit. On your first appointment, you'll be drained of some of your bodily fluids like pee, blood, and cervical juice (a pap smear). From these fluids, your doctor will test you for German measles, hepatitis B, and chicken pox. You'll also be given a CBC, and STS, and tested for HIV and STDs. But don't fear, it'll all be done PDQ (pretty darn quick) and you should be A-OK (I'll let you figure that one out for yourself). Your pee will be examined for bacteria, sugar, and albumin. Your blood pressure will be tested and charted. Some of these tests will be repeated during every doctor's visit throughout your pregnancy.

Assuming you pass the first round of tests, you can start cramming for your glucose screen. You don't want to fail that one or you'll have to take a three-hour glucose tolerance exam that's a killer. There's also a vaginal and rectal test for Group B streptococcus. And don't forget your triple screen blood test at about sixteen weeks. This will test for increased risk for Down syndrome and spinal cord abnormalities. There may be also be a test for Tay-Sachs, sickle cell, or any number of other genetic conditions. And, for extra credit, there's the optional CVS or amniocentesis.

And finally, on graduation day, after you've delivered your thesis (a.k.a. your child), you will be awarded an important document worthy of framing. This piece of paper will be your baby's birth certificate, showing that you've passed all tests necessary to hold the position of "Parent." You'll serve in that position for your entire life and work long grueling hours with no overtime, pension, or even a decent health plan.

After your baby is born, the tests will continue. In fact, there will be years' worth of tests that you'll have to endure. But this time the tests won't be given by a medical professional; they'll be given by your own child who will forever be testing your patience and limitations. So, good luck out there. Study well and *E Pluribus Unum*.

Dreams and Other Nightmares

Being pregnant is an emotional time, and like any other mental anguish, it's going to show up in your dreams. I'm not talking about beautiful dreams like running through a meadow holding your halo-headed newborn. I'm talking about weird, freakish, and often disturbing dreams.

At the early stages of my pregnancy, most of my dreams centered on me causing my child extreme harm. I would dream that I left it at a mall. Or that I would forget to feed it for days at a time. I once dreamed that I was at the beach during the hottest day of the year, and I suddenly remembered that I had left my child locked in the trunk of the car. Panicked, I rushed to the parking lot and opened the trunk. I found my tiny loved one shriveled up like one of the pod people in *Cocoon*.

About halfway though my pregnancy, my dreams started to change. Instead of centering around my being the worst mother in the world, they were about how deformed my newborn was. By far the most disturbing dream I had was the one where my child was born without any skin. I wasn't so much disturbed by her lack of skin as I was terrified of telling my husband about it. I remember holding my slimy little infant fearing that my husband would come into the room and get really mad at me.

In another dream, I was trying to breastfeed my baby, but it was having trouble latching on. I looked down only to find that my child was born with a beak. I had several other dreams where my child was deformed. Once it had a severe wandering eye. Another time it had a face full of hair.

I'm no psychiatrist, but it's not hard to figure out that being pregnant is incredibly scary. You may appear calm and steady during the daytime, but at night, your fear, along with your imaginary child, will rear its ugly head. But don't worry. These are only dreams, not premonitions. Despite all of my nighttime horror shows, my child was born without a beak or extra facial hair. So when you experience one of your nightmares, just relax and enjoy the show.

To Tell or Not to Tell

Now that you're pregnant, you want to shout it out to the world! It's by far the most exciting news that you've ever had! You can't wait to tell your friends, your family, and every member of your high school graduation class. I understand completely. I too was excited, and couldn't wait to share the news. But as you know, people advise you to wait until the second trimester before you start telling people, because the risk of miscarriage decreases significantly at that time.

Although I knew in my head that telling someone I was pregnant was not going to make my embryo dislodge from my womb, why take a chance? We agreed to hold off blabbing about it for a while. But that wasn't as easy as I expected. Whenever a friend asked me what was new, I bit my tongue. Soon, my tongue had so many holes I could drain spaghetti with it.

I felt as if I were going to burst with excitement. I was like an overinflated tire. If I didn't spill the beans soon and alleviate some of the pressure, I was going to pop. So, for the sake of highway safety I decided to tell someone. I decided that a relative stranger would be the perfect someone. Telling a stranger the good news would be like that five-second rule about eating dropped food—it doesn't really count.

Soon after my decision, I saw my eighty-five-year-old neighbor, Grace, walk past my house. Grace would be perfect. She's not a friend or a family member; she's just someone who lives in my neighborhood. Grace has hip trouble so once a day she takes a slow walk around the block. And man, do I mean slow. By the time she gets home, it's almost time for her to go around again.

When she walked past me this time, she greeted me with her usual remark, "Hi, dear, what's new?" And finally, I spilled the beans! I told her about being pregnant and how excited I was. I babbled on and on about what my husband did when I told him and how sick I was feeling. It was so good to finally share the news! Grace looked at me, smiled and said, "Is that a new blouse, dear?" I realized then that Grace may have some hearing trouble as well, but I didn't care. I finally told someone.

After Grace, I was able to keep quiet for some time, but found that it was really hard to keep news (and a belly) of that size hidden. In addition to a thickening waistline, there were several other signs that got people suspicious. But, like any good pregnant woman in her first trimester, I lied. If I yawned a great deal, I told people I had stayed up for Letterman. Passing on wine meant I had too much to drink the night before. If I declined coffee at the office, I told coworkers I had a pot's worth at home. Nausea at a family dinner meant I had Indian food for lunch, and my comically large breasts meant I was about to get my period. I realized that I was an incredibly good liar and fabricated tales as only the Brothers Grimm could do.

Now, I'm not suggesting that you keep your mouth shut during this exciting time. It's a very personal decision. You may be too superstitious to consider tempting fate with the news. Or you may be too much of a blabbermouth to conceal it. But, whether you do or don't decide to start sharing the good news, I have some words of pregnancy wisdom to share with you (see, I told you I had a hard time keeping my mouth shut):

1. If you do decide to tell people, be picky. I feel that you should tell only the close friends and relatives you would turn to for comfort in difficult times. In case you do suffer a miscarriage, you'll no doubt tell them anyway because you'll need their shoulders to cry on.

2. Have a list of premade excuses about why you're abstaining from alcohol, cigarettes, and coffee, and while you're at it, include one for why you can't stop yawning all day. You may find that you're not as talented a liar as I am, and it may be hard to come up with excuses on the spot.

3. If you feel as if you're going to burst with excitement as I did and you have to tell just one person, I suggest that you tell your boss (if you feel comfortable enough). Your work may slack off for a while, and you'll want to protect yourself. You may be preoccupied, moody, tired, and nauseated. You'll be on the phone making doctor's appointments and will surf the Internet for pregnancy info. You'll be so elated with the miracle growing in your belly that such a mundane thing as earning a living may lose its importance.

4. Tell any and all pregnant women. You'll be amazed at what saying "I'm pregnant too" will do. Instantly, the bond will form. You'll share your fears, your excitement, your advice, and of course, your belly size (this will soon become as big a comparison issue as men in locker rooms).

You'll find other "preggos" an amazing source of some much-needed support.

Pregnancy Math

Remember your old math classes in school? You memorized formulas, studied graphs, and figured out equations like how fast train A would pass train B if it were the third Tuesday of the month in a leap year. You'd put your head in your hand in frustration and ponder the age-old question: "When will I ever use this stuff?" Well, it turns out that the time has finally come.

From the moment you conceive, you're going to need basic math skills. You'll either be trying to calculate how far along you are, or to figure out your due date. To the naive, you conceive a child and give birth nine months later. But to the educated, it's not that simple. In fact, figuring out basic pregnancy equations can be more complicated than figuring out the train one.

For pregnancy doesn't start the moment the sperm penetrates the egg like your mom told you during that uncomfortable "birds and bees" talk. Miraculously, you become pregnant on the first day of your last period. At least that's the case from an O.B.'s point of view. The theory is based on the fact that no woman is quite sure of the day that she ovulated (unless of course she was as neurotic as me and used an ovulation predictor kit), but she usually remembers when she began her last period. So, the nine-month countdown begins on that date. It's like getting extra pregnancy weeks for free. It's sort of the baker's dozen of gestation.

Now, since a full-term pregnancy lasts for forty weeks, you're actually two weeks pregnant when you conceive, and about a month along when you're finally aware that you're pregnant. Pretty cool, huh?

Some women like to base their gestation on ten four-week intervals. It makes calculating much easier, but it changes the standard nine-month gestation into ten, and that's already too confusing. I won't discuss that theory any further without at least a prerequisite knowledge of logarithms. Luckily, the vast majority of preggies go by the nine-month, forty-week standard.

Now, it's time for the pop quiz: How many months pregnant would you be if you were entering your third trimester? Well, let's see . . . it seems simple enough. Each trimester is three months long, so you'd be starting your seventh month. Right? Wrong! All trimesters are not considered equal. The first trimester is the longest with fourteen weeks, and the second trimester is only twelve. So, if you were entering your third trimester you'd be twenty-six weeks pregnant and since there are 4.3 weeks in the average month, you'd be how many months pregnant?! Who knows? Who cares? The whole thing is too confusing. So, I have an idea.

I suggest that all you keep track of is how many weeks pregnant you are and keep it at that. Don't worry about months. Not only does this make the countdown to delivery simple (forty weeks minus "X" weeks pregnant equals delivery), but it forces others to do the math for you. When someone stops you in the checkout line and asks you how far along you are, tell them that you're twenty-three weeks. Then the fun starts as their eyes glaze over in frustration trying to calculate twenty-three weeks into months.

Not only is my "weeks" theory more convenient, but it's good practice for when the baby finally comes out. You'll notice that a baby is never a month-and-a-half old, it's always six weeks. Never a year-and-a-half, but rather eighteen months. Not until your tot is two years old do you revert back to the rest of the world's twelve-month calendar year.

How to Eat for Two

No, this is not a segment about nutrition. I don't know the first thing about beta-carotines or triglycerides. The most scientific sounding food I ingest is Häagen-Dazs. But I do know a thing or two about the dynamics of pregnancy eating.

The first dynamic is what I call the "I Have to Eat Now!" syndrome. I know you've experienced the hunger sensation before you conceived. Your tummy would growl and you'd be a little lightheaded. But you don't know hunger till you've experienced pregnancy hunger. All of a sudden you turn into the "Feed Me" plant from *Little Shop of Horrors*. Your body is burning a lot of calories to make this baby, and your metabolism is changing. Because of this, your blood sugar will drop like the price of tech stocks during the crash.

When you experience one of these blood sugar drops, you'll need to eat and you'll need to eat fast! You'll invade your kitchen like locust on corn. Anything will do. Raw hot dogs, frozen peas, even powdered cake mix. Soon, your blood sugar will stabilize and you can rest. You'll catch a glimpse of your reflection in the toaster and see the face of a crazed animal after devouring a zebra carcass.

There are a few things to do to avoid this scene from a *National Geographic* special:

1. Try not to have an empty stomach. Eat a lot of little meals throughout the day.
2. Keep healthy snacks available—a bag of trail mix in your purse, some peanut butter crackers in your office drawer, and so forth.
3. Eat protein instead of sugar. Protein takes longer to digest and fills your stomach for a longer period.

The second dynamic of pregnancy eating is cravings. Suddenly, you'll have a strong desire for a certain kind of food. It may be one of your favorite foods or one that's grossed you out in the past. It's all a crap shoot. Not all pregnant women suffer with cravings to the same degree, but almost every one of them will experience some type of noshing urge.

Personally, I never had the kind of intense cravings that I saw on TV. I wished that I would have. Nothing would have pleased me more than to send my husband out during a blizzard to fetch me some turkey jerky. But my cravings were never that strong and besides, we live in Southern California. Still, it would have been the *least* he could have done, considering my condition.

As with almost everything else in the world of pregnancy ailments, cravings are caused by hormones, which should stabilize around the third or fourth month. And as your hormones stabilize, so will your cravings. You'll still have them, but they won't be as intense.

Believe it or not, cravings actually serve a purpose. When you get an urge for a particular kind of food, it means that your body needs it for some purpose. You may be nutritionally depleted in some area or need something to help with nausea, and cravings let you know about it. I found that most of my cravings revolved around protein. I found myself eating loads of meat, chicken, and milk shakes (they have protein, don't they?). It seems that every day your baby takes vitamins and minerals from you that it needs to survive. Yes, that embryo that you adore is basically a tick sucking away your life force. So go ahead and eat. If you have a hankering for some kind of food, and it's not going to harm your precious parasite, by all means, scarf it down.

Chapter Two

The Second Month

One down, eight more to go! I know that one month isn't much in terms of gestation, but it was plenty of time for me to learn the number one rule of pregnancy: Don't complain! I remember my second month as a blur of nausea. But whenever I uttered a word of despair, people glared at me, their eyes filled with disappointment and shock. I learned my lesson quickly that discussing pregnancy misery is thought to be unwomanly. Maybe even sinful.

I know what they were thinking. That here I was, being given one of the greatest gifts a woman can receive, and all I could do was complain. Well . . . they were right. But just because you're given a nice gift doesn't mean that it's necessarily "you." Don't get me wrong. I know how lucky I was to be able to conceive and give birth to a healthy beautiful baby. I don't take that for granted for one minute. But I learned an important lesson from Mike Brady, who told his daughter Jan: "Find something that you're good at, and be good at it," and the thing that I'm quite good at doing is complaining. And being pregnant gave me so many opportunities to use my God-given talent.

Whenever I discussed my body's increased state of woe, people said "Aw, c'mon, it's not really that bad. Besides, look what you're getting in return."

Yes, I knew that I was getting a baby in return for my grief, but it still didn't seem fair. How come being blessed with a child meant having to suffer through so much discomfort? It's like being offered a great promotion at work that's conditional on a bout of Montezuma's revenge. Sure, you're grateful for the promotion, but should one be expected to *enjoy* the cramping and diarrhea?

In the scheme of things, I didn't have that unusual a pregnancy. I was never hospitalized for morning sickness. I wasn't bedridden for months at a time. I never got hemorrhoids or toxemia. I didn't even poop on the delivery room table (or so I choose to believe). But even without these experiences, I consider my pregnancy to be a miserable journey, and this first trimester to be the worst trek.

If you're not experiencing morning sickness by now, chances are that you're not going to be. For whatever cosmic reason, your body will bypass this horrific aspect of pregnancy. You are the gold medal winner of the Olympic Games of procreation. But be warned, there are many more games to be played. And, in the words of Caesar, "Let the games begin!"

Hell Hath No Fury Like a Woman with Child

We've all seen the stereotypical pregnant woman portrayed in movies. She can go from angel to devil with one fallopian tube tied behind her back. In real life, things are much different. There is no "angel" stage of a mood swing. At least there wasn't for me.

❝ I didn't know I was pregnant. All I knew was that everything my husband did bugged the hell out of me. When I found out, I was so happy to be pregnant and not headed for divorce court. **❞**
—Beverly

It's pretty safe to assume that whenever a mood hits, you'll become quite an unpleasant person. It's not surprising though. It's hard to feel all warm and fuzzy when you lie in bed moaning in morning sickness agony. Just like morning sickness, the mood swings that hit during pregnancy hit hard and fast. They're very similar to PMS in that they're both caused by hormones. But if PMS is like the irritating sound of a jackhammer, pregnancy mood swings are like that jackhammer pounding away during a heavy metal concert.

As sick as you are with morning sickness, you'll no doubt manage to have enough energy to pull off several mood swings. You'll probably get upset with your husband over anything and everything. Either he isn't being considerate, or he's being too considerate, which is even worse.

I have two bits of advice, one for you and one for the horrid beast you may now refer to as your husband. For you, I suggest that you make a blanket apology to cover any atrocious words that may spew from your lips in the upcoming months. For him: leave her alone whenever possible. And for God's sake, don't just discount your wife's attitude as a mood swing. Remember what used to happen when you told her she was cranky because she had PMS? It's going to get her even more upset now. If you feel you must speak, don't argue, don't react, don't say anything at all except, "Yes, dear" or "Whatever you say, dear." My husband repeated these phrases so often that it became second nature. I'm tempted to tell him that he doesn't have to say them so often anymore, but then again, why ruin a good thing?

Your Superhero Nose

A funny thing happened to me on my way to becoming pregnant. I became a superhero. Or at least I developed a superhero's sense of smell. Just as Superman can leap tall buildings in a single bound, I could smell small bulldogs at the local pound. One day, I opened my front door and was able to smell Chinese food cooking from a restaurant several blocks away. Same restaurant. Same location. Superhero nose.

I don't know why it happens, but for some strange reason, every pregnant woman develops a superhuman sense of smell. It's like the *Gilligan's Island* episode where the castaways eat radioactive food that intensifies their senses. One of them eats carrots and can see a ship miles off shore. If I had been on the island, I could have smelled the varnish on the poop deck.

It may sound like a cool thing to experience, sort of like being able to lift a car over your head during an emergency, but most times, this talent for smelling isn't at all enjoyable.

"I thought my husband was having an affair because he'd come home smelling of perfume. He's a high school teacher and said that some of his students must be wearing it. Even though I believed him, he made his kids promise never to wear perfume until I delivered.**"**
—Allison

It is actually quite awful. You take a woman who is nauseated by the mere thought of food, and give her the power to smell every meal cooking in the neighborhood. It is yet another cruel trick of Mother Nature.

I have no advice on how to lessen your sense of smell (short of clamping a clothespin on your nose), but I will point out some interesting advantages:

1. You can kiss your husband hello when he comes home from work, and tell him what he had for lunch that day.
2. You can walk past your coworker and notice that she's changed her brand of fabric softener.
3. You could get a job sniffing luggage for drugs at your local international airport.
4. You can offer your assistance to rescue teams scaling mountains and hillsides looking for missing hikers.

Pregnancy Junkie

As soon as it was official that the rabbit had died, I headed down to the local bookstore to get some reading material. Since I had never been pregnant before, there had to be a few things to learn. I bought the basic bibles. I got a book about what happens to the baby each week, each month, even each day. I got a picture book of a baby growing inside the mommy and a picture book of a mommy growing with a baby inside of her. I got books from my doctor and books from my friends. I became a pregnancy book junkie. I couldn't read enough about what was going on inside me.

When there were no more books left to read, I went on the Internet. I found a chat room where I conversed with other preggies. I found a Web site that gave me a daily breakdown of what my kid was doing. I knew the day my baby developed its fingerprints, and celebrated when it took its first pee in my amniotic fluid. My head was filled with facts and figures. I could have been awarded an honorary degree in obstetrics from Harvard University.

But like a true junkie, I hit rock bottom. I would look at the same books two or three times a day. I couldn't have a twinge without cross-referencing book after book until I made my diagnosis. I was out of control. Soon, my friends wouldn't listen to me. My parents found me boring. My husband couldn't ask how I was doing without me going on and on about my increased blood level or cholesterol count.

But in the end, these books gave me comfort and that was the important thing. They were like my owner's manual for the greatest household addition we ever got. And they will also come in handy if I ever decide to get pregnant again (yeah, right).

If you're like me, I have a few suggestions on where you can go to get your fix. The bookstore is the most obvious place. I was astounded by the amount of coverage given to this common condition. There are books written by doctors, therapists, psychologists, even celebrities. It seems anyone with a medical license or a Screen Actor's Guild card is qualified to get in on the picture.

If you're computer literate, I suggest the Web. My favorite place was *www.pregnancycalendar.com*. There, you can type some of your relevant pregnancy info and get a personalized calendar with the day-to-day progress of your fetus's development. It's absolutely fascinating and I suggest you check it out. I also liked *www.pregnancyfit.com*. It's full of advice on health and nutrition that I found useful. Also go to *www.ivillage.com*. It's particularly good if you want to talk with other pregnant woman to compare and contrast your situation. But do your own surfing. There are hundreds of sites that you can explore.

Television is another place to turn. Cable channels are chock-full of shows like *A Baby Story*, *Pregnancy for Dummies*, or *Birthday*. On any given week, turn to the Discovery Channel or the Health Channel for your fill of ultrasounds, placentas, and mucus plugs. Now that's "must see" TV!

If you don't get cable, head to your local video store and check out movies like *Nine Months*, *She's Having My Baby*, or *Junior*. They may not be completely accurate from a medical point of view (like the fact that Arnold Schwartzenegger is the one carrying the child), but they'll do. Anything will do. That's how you know you're a true addict.

Spotting

There's this saying that I've always loved. It was meant to describe war, but I always use it to describe airplane travel: hours of boredom interrupted by brief moments of terror. I've altered it a bit for pregnancy. I now say: hours of discomfort interrupted by brief moments of terror. One of those brief moments is called *spotting*.

Spotting is when some blood passes through your vagina. You usually discover it on one of your many journeys to the bathroom to pee. You wipe yourself and the toilet paper is streaked with blood. Your heart stops as you think the worst. You're losing your baby!

But put your mind to rest. Spotting, although terrifying, happens in more than 25 percent of all pregnancies. Although it's more frequent in the first trimester, it can happen at any time. Spotting can either be limited to a single drop of blood, or it can be a steady stream for a couple of hours. It can range from a brownish color to bright red.

I spotted several times during the first trimester, and then once again in the last. At first, I too was panicked. But my O.B. put my mind at ease. After time, I would see a spot or two on my underpants and think nothing of it. In fact, it became fun. It was like an undergarment Rorschach test. Once the drops of blood formed together to create the spitting image of Elvis. I thought of shellacking the panties and sending them off to Graceland, but then I thought it best just to throw them in the wash.

You should tell your doctor if you notice some spotting for the first time, or definitely if the spotting continues to flow for more than a couple of hours or is accompanied by cramps. He may want you to come to the office for an ultrasound so that he can determine where the spotting is coming from. Is the placenta burrowing into the lining of the uterus? Is there some kind of irritation to the cervix? There are many reasons for the blood other than a miscarriage, but only your doctor can tell for sure.

By the way, if you do need to see the doctor, there's no need to bring any blood-soaked napkins or panties in with you unless he instructs you to do so. You may think me silly for even mentioning this, but some women do it. I know a woman who brought in her bloody pads that she'd wrapped in foil and placed in an airtight freezer bag. The doctor thought she was giving him homemade baked goods. Not only won't your doctor be able to tell anything from your pads, but chances are, he'll be pretty grossed out. Even a doctor has limitations.

Once your doctor examines you and puts your mind at ease, he'll send you on your merry way with one warning: No sex until you stop spotting for seven days. And if you ever do spot again, you'll find that you won't panic so much. Who knows, you may even have your own celebrity spotting.

I Need to Lie Down

During the first trimester you're tired all the time. It's no wonder since your body is so hard at work. Just think of the tremendous amount of energy it uses to make a baby. I get tired just making dinner. So pamper your body and treat it well. If it needs more rest, by all means, give it more.

Unlike the fatigue that you'll experience during the other trimesters, you have an enormous advantage now. You can actually sleep if you want to. You should savor these days when you can sleep long and hard for they will soon come to an end. In the second trimester your belly will be so big you'll have to sleep on your side. And by your third, your heartburn will be so bad that you'll have to sleep in a chair. But I'll fill you in on those things later on. I don't want to give any of the good stuff away.

My best advice is . . . get used to it! Having a kid is exhausting whether it's on the inside of you or the outside. You'll crave a nap when your child is learning to sleep through the night. Then while he's teething. Then during night traumas, and ear infections, and monsters in the closet, and so on and so on until it's the senior prom when you're up all night waiting for him to come home while he's out doing God knows what. Ooops. There I go again, giving the good stuff away.

Oh My Achin' Head

In addition to all the other joyous side effects of pregnancy, you may also experience a lot of headaches. You may not be aware of this headache connection, but it's true. You may think, why headaches anyway? What does my brain have to do in order to make a baby in my uterus? Well, it's not your brain that's the trouble; rather it's your hormones causing all the subcranial pounding. In addition to everyday headaches, changes in hormone levels bring on more sinus headaches and migraines as well.

When I started getting my headaches, I was opposed to taking any kind of medication even though my obstetrician said I could take Tylenol (or any other form of acetaminophen). I was a purist. I didn't want to take anything that might cause me to give birth to a child with three kneecaps. So when my head hurt I decided to take the natural approach. I relaxed in a dark room with scented candles. I put a cold compress on my forehead. I ate a snack or took a long walk. I tried everything I could think of to stop the incessant pain. Finally, I did one thing that made all the difference in the world. I changed my mind about taking Tylenol.

I had never ridden out a headache before being pregnant, and I can tell you it ain't pretty. I, like most of you who have had a headache, would simply pop a couple of pills and say good-bye to pain. But, without those glorious gelcaps, a headache can linger and linger and linger. Sometimes I would go to sleep with a headache and wake up with it the next morning. And sometimes, even the morning after that! I never fully appreciated a good painkiller until I conceived.

I'm pretty sure that most doctors will let you take Tylenol (and some may prescribe something stronger if you have a severe headache or migraine), but I would definitely ask that question when you're interviewing obstetricians. To me, believing in over-the-counter medication is a more important qualification in an O.B. than actually passing medical school.

"Urine" for Fun

I'm sure that there are some of you out there who think that incessant peeing is a joy reserved only for pregnant women in their last trimester. Well, surprise! You get to enjoy it during the first trimester as well.

You probably had no idea of this lovely side effect since the embryo doesn't seem big enough to press down on your bladder. The little thing couldn't weigh more than a wad of gum. But even though it doesn't weigh much, it seems that your uterus is growing nonetheless and that's what's pushing into your bladder. On top of that, as a pregnant woman, you have a lot more blood and other bodily fluids coursing through your veins, so there is a greater liquid turnover rate.

Although I can't stop your constant desire to excrete, I can offer a bit of insight with regard to the peeing milieu:

1. First, in case of a peeing emergency, become familiar with the bathroom situation whenever you enter a new place. This is similar to knowing the exit routes in case of a fire.

2. Use night-lights. Put up one in the bathroom and, if needed, several more marking the way to get there. You'll find that you may need to pee several times during the night and I found it best not to turn on any lights. Not because you might awaken your spouse (no need to worry about making *his* life easier when you're pregnant), but because turning on a bright light in a dark room is shocking to your system and could interfere with your ability to put yourself back to sleep after you're done peeing.

3. If you decided not to tell your coworkers that you're pregnant, be prepared to be a subject for the rumor mill. Running off to the bathroom a dozen times a day may make your officemates think that you've taken up an illegal habit.

Miscarriage

The biggest fear during the first trimester is miscarriage. The fact is that about 20 to 30 percent of all pregnancies will end in one, depending on the woman's age (precise numbers are difficult to determine because some women who miscarry very early never knew they were pregnant). I know that's not a comforting statistic now, but if you do experience a miscarriage, it may give you some comfort to know that they are so common. At least it did for me.

I had a miscarriage several months before I got pregnant with the child that I have now. I was in my second month and one night I started getting very small cramps. They felt like tiny menstrual cramps. By the next morning these small cramps were a little bit stronger. I knew something wasn't right, but like most potentially bad things, I dealt with the situation by denial and rationalization. It wasn't until I started to bleed that I rushed to the doctor in hysterics.

The doctor gave me an ultrasound, took some blood, and told me that he'd call me with the results. That afternoon, he told me that the blood tests came back, and that my blood levels were decreasing. My pregnancy was terminating. My child—and my dreams—were dead.

The news hit me with such a deep sadness that I couldn't control the tears. And just as my emotional pain peaked, the physical pain began. The mild cramping that I had denied suddenly became extremely painful. And the slight bleeding that I had that morning was now a torrential downpour. The doctor prescribed a painkiller and told me I would bleed for about a week.

And bleed I did. There was more blood than in a Rambo movie. And it wasn't like menstrual blood, it was packed full of clots. Every time I went to the bathroom I was constantly reminded of the miscarriage. I would look at the clumps in the toilet bowl and think of what might have been, "That might have been a forearm," or "This could have been a shoulder." Every time I went to the bathroom, and flushed away more potential body parts, it brought the whole experience back.

Because I wasn't that far along, I didn't require any medical intervention. But, if you're over roughly eight to ten weeks pregnant, there might be enough developed tissue in your uterus to warrant having a dilation and curettage (a "D and C"). You're given a drug to relax you; then a doctor dilates your cervix and cleans out the walls of your uterus. Afterwards, you'll have to be driven home and sent to bed. You'll experience some cramping and bleeding, but all in all, it won't be all that painful, physically anyway.

There's a new drug on the market called Misoprostol that may provide you with an option other than a D and C. If it's determined that your pregnancy isn't viable, but your body hasn't begun to miscarry on its own, Misoprostol can help. It causes your uterus to contract and expel the potentially infectious tissue on its own, thereby saving you from having to undergo any medical procedure.

If you do suffer a miscarriage, be kind to yourself and, if possible, avoid contact with others for a while. I had my

> **"I felt so deflated. Even though we'd only known that I was pregnant for a couple of weeks, we were so excited about it. It's amazing how quickly you can fall in love with something."**
> —My sister, Laurie, who had a miscarriage while I was writing this book

mom call all the people who knew that I was pregnant and tell them what happened. After the weekend passed I was able to start talking about what happened, and I suggest that you wait until you're good and ready. I found that even though talking about it helped, many people were ignorantly insensitive. "It's for the best" or "Don't worry, you can have another one" were the most commonly offered well-intentioned but unkind words of wisdom. I'd wonder how they would feel if I said the same thing to them about someone they'd lost. Eventually, I started off each conversation by saying, "I know there's nothing to say, so don't say anything." People meant well, but they could be quite clueless.

Unfortunately, after a miscarriage, you can't just jump back on that proverbial horse and try again. You'll need to wait until after your next period to have unprotected sex again. This will give the lining of your uterus enough time to rebuild itself. If you were neurotic about conceiving before the miscarriage, you'll probably be even more neurotic now. And once you conceive again (and you will), you'll be frantic about every little twinge. Was that a cramp? Oh my God, there's blood! I can't tell you to relax because I know that I sure couldn't.

Although I don't have a solution to miscarriages, I do know one thing about them that's certain. *There is nothing that you could have done to cause a miscarriage, or to prevent it from happening.* I know that part of you feels that you must have done something wrong. But try as much as you can to put that thought out of your mind because it simply is not true.

If you do have a miscarriage, my heart goes out to you. But just like other tragedies, time is a great healer. It's been over a year since I went through mine and even though I remember the events with complete clarity, the painful feelings have faded. And now I can see that if I didn't lose the first child, I never would have given birth to the one I have now. And, for me, that would have been the greatest tragedy of all.

Sex During the First Trimester

Sex during pregnancy is very much like Jello 1-2-3 (a reference that only those well into their thirties will understand). There are three completely distinct layers that go along with each trimester. Because of this, I'm going to discuss each of these different layers with you, in each of the three trimesters that they go with.

Although I was never in the bedrooms of pregnant women during their first trimester, I can't imagine that it was a very active room. What with all the nausea, headaches, irritability, and achy breasts, I don't think many of these women were in the mood for much lovin'.

Every book and every doctor I know say that sex is fine when you're pregnant, provided you are not having a high-risk pregnancy. They say it doesn't harm the embryo in any way, but, in my pregnancy induced, overly cautious state of mind, I couldn't see how first trimester sex would be very good for it either. I mean, the first trimester is the most influential one in the child's development. It's the time when crucial cells are dividing that will one day become the internal organs, the skeleton, or the skin. I would have felt mighty guilty if my kid emerged with a spleen dangling from its chin just because I wanted a night of action.

As it turned out, first trimester sex wasn't even an option for me—doctor's orders. Because I had the miscarriage, he instructed me to have complete pelvic rest. Pelvic rest is the medical term for "no sex." Your vagina has become like the White House; nothing is getting in there without proper clearance. I can't say that I was all that disappointed to hear the news since I was feeling pretty sick as it was. Now, with the abstinence orders, my husband wasn't feeling too well himself. If you had a miscarriage before, and your doctor tells you that it's okay to have sex, that's fine. Many doctors feel differently than mine did.

If your doctor tells you that all systems are go, and if all your systems feel like going, then by all means, go ahead. But if you're feeling rather unfrisky, tell your hubby about the complete pelvic rest thing. Tell him that it's doctor's orders. Sure, maybe not your doctor, but a doctor nonetheless.

Chapter Three

The Third Month

*F*ace it. You're a mess. You're constipated, cranky, and congested. And those are only the "C"s. I can't tell you when all of these pregnancy side effects will end. In fact, some are only going to get worse. But, I can tell you one incredible thing. It's probably the most wonderful thing that you've heard in a long time. Your morning sickness will probably start to go away by the end of this month! I know that you don't believe it, but for the vast majority of you, it will happen. It won't happen in a day. It will happen gradually. It might get better, only to get worse again. And then, finally it will end.

For me, it was a McDonald's Big N' Tasty Burger that turned things around. I was in one of my "I'm so hungry, I can eat your face" kind of moods and my husband and I went out for a burger. My sesame seed–coated piece of heaven went down as smoothly as twelve-year-old Scotch, and stayed down with no trouble at all! To this day, I still order those burgers. I gobble them down with a smile on my face and a prayer in my heart for all of the poor pregnant women all over the world.

In this month, your baby will change from an embryo to a fetus. Then it's only a matter of time. Soon it'll be a newborn, infant, toddler, kid, teen, adult, and then an occasional visitor whenever a home-cooked meal or clean laundry is needed. During the third month, your baby will develop eyelids and fingers. Also, its anal membrane will become perforated! Now, doesn't that bring a tear of joy to your eye?

I hope that the third month will go by quickly for you and that your morning sickness will start to subside. But while you're waiting, your pregnancy hormones are kicking into higher gear this month. Because of this, there are some more goodies to look forward to. So sit back, relax, and enjoy the coming attractions.

I Can't Breathe!

Just as your body makes a lot more blood when you're pregnant, it also makes a lot more snot. I have no idea why a body would do this, what reason it could have for making an abundant amount of mucus, but I'm sure it knows best.

It's quite frustrating that as soon as the morning sickness starts to pass, when each day was like having the flu, now comes the congestion, when each day is like having a cold.

❝ One night while I was sleeping my husband got out of bed. I woke up and asked him what was wrong, and he said he was going to close the window because there's a sick cat outside. But as soon as I woke up, it stopped. It turns out he heard me snoring. **❞**

—Nancy

And just like a cold, pregnancy congestion always seems to get worse at night. My husband said that I even started to snore. This made me extremely happy since he snores—I could finally get even. At last he would know how frustrating it is to sleep with the lulling sound of construction noise going on at the next pillow. But I never got my revenge because I discovered something even more irritating about him than his snoring. His ability to sleep through someone else's snoring while he continues to snore the whole time. Life isn't fair.

Pregnancy congestion is just like the congestion that's associated with a common cold. And since no one has found a cure for a cold yet, don't look to me for an answer. I can, however, suggest a few things that may help you breathe just a little bit easier:

1. Use an antihistamine like Sudafed, Dimetapp Extend Tabs, Chlor-Trimeton, or Benadryl. Check with your doctor first and if he gives the okay, have him recommend a dosage. It may be different than that specified on the label.

2. Stock up on saline spray. It'll keep your nose moist, which may not make sense, but it works. I know you think you want to dry out your nose, but trust me, this way is best.

3. Alternate hot and cold compresses over your sinuses. Again, this helps to open up the passages.

4. Sleep with your head elevated. That way you keep the snot rolling downhill.

5. Rub Vicks Vaporub. Not only will it help you breathe easier, but it'll bring back memories of your childhood, which can be pretty comforting at a time like this.

6. Turn on the humidifier. Once again, it'll add moisture to the air and therefore your nose. Yes, it doesn't make sense, but again, trust me. I'm a mom now and I know best.

7. Sport those nasal strips like the athletes wear. They're

Band-Aids for the bridge of your nose that open the airways and allow you to breathe better. They can also relieve some of your snoring, which will make your husband sleep better (as if you care).

Is My Baby Okay in There?

You already know that parents worry about their children. Are they eating right? Are they having trouble in school? Have they found Daddy's special videotape collection? But did you know that parental worrying begins even before a child is born? From the moment of conception, mothers and even the fathers worry about their in utero baby. In utero worrying is even more frustrating than "out utero" worrying because you can't check on the kid yet. Your doctor may assure you that all is fine in there, but it's still hard to believe it without seeing for yourself. A part of me used to wish that my baby needed a small operation so they'd be forced to pull it out of my tummy for just a minute so I could take a peek. Nothing major mind you, just an overgrown toenail that needed tending to.

Your worries may be irrational, but even irrational fears feel real. One of my big worries was that the child I was carrying around in my belly wasn't even human. When I was about two months pregnant, I saw an article in *Life* magazine that showed the fetus of a pig, a simian, and a human, all at the same stage in their gestation period. The three embryos looked almost identical. It wasn't until the specific pig, simian, or human DNA took over that the blob got a nose or a snout. I was thoroughly convinced that my fetus's DNA wasn't working properly and I was carrying around something closer to *Babe* than baby.

You may also worry that your kid isn't still alive in there.

I mean, you can't feel it kicking yet. There were many times during my pregnancy that I thought my baby had bitten the big one. I was sure that it was floating around at the top of my uterus like a dead goldfish in a bowl. If it's old enough, (about 10 to 12 weeks) your O.B. can use a fetal heart monitor to hear its heart beating. This should reassure you. But still, there is a long time in between appointments. What do you do while you wait?

There's a chance that if your doctor can pick up the baby's heartbeat, maybe you can too. Through the Internet, your local baby shop, or even discount department store, you can rent or purchase a Doppler fetal heart monitor similar to that used by your doctor. Be sure to read the directions carefully, and be patient. Your baby is quite small and your tummy's quite large (no offense). It's common that you may not even find the heartbeat the first time you try. Don't panic. Don't make deals with God. Just wait a few days and try again. Soon your baby's heartbeat should come in loud and clear, and give yours a chance to stop beating so fast.

And with time, you can rest assured that, despite your concerns, your baby's doing just fine.

Here I Grow Again

I have a theory about weight gain during pregnancy. I believe that there's one crucial factor that will determine whether you'll carry like you swallowed a baseball, or the entire team. That factor is the length of your waist.

I have an extremely short waist, which I blame for the majority of my pregnancy complaints, as well as my difficulty in buying well-fitting jeans. If you have a short waist, there's nowhere for the baby to go but out. By the end of my third month I outgrew my husband's clothes, and by the end of the

❝ I forecast the weather on the local news, and because I gained so much weight, they had to shrink the map of the United States. It seemed that whenever I stood in front of it, I blocked the entire eastern seaboard. **❞**
—Jeannette

sixth month, I outgrew the car cover. By the end of my pregnancy, my child no longer had the luxury of being in the fetal position. The poor thing had to be curled up like a cinnamon roll. I was so big my obstetrician actually asked me if I had a history of giants in my family. Was I carrying a kid or a Dodge Caravan?

My theory is that if you're blessed with a long waist, you'll have far fewer pregnancy complaints. You'll have less heartburn, less indigestion, and less belly, for a longer period of time. There's so much room from your breasts to your crotch if you're long-waisted, that your baby can more or less stand on tippy-toes for its entire gestation.

It is recommended that a pregnant woman should gain between 25 and 35 pounds. I felt confident that I'd be closer to the 25-pound range. I'm a short person, only 5'3" if I'm wearing thick socks. So when I packed on my extra 40 pounds, I was disgusted with myself. I would have been okay if I hadn't been pregnant around Christmastime, for it was then that I was surrounded by my favorite food group: gift baskets.

It's too bad that I didn't watch my weight gain more carefully because two weeks after I gave birth, I had dropped 22 pounds, over half the weight that I had gained. If I hadn't indulged, I would have been back to my normal weight in a matter of weeks, just like the girls on *Baywatch*.

The way you'll gain weight will probably be similar to the way most preggos do. At first, your boobs will start to grow . . . and grow and grow and grow. They'll become the "Jack and the Beanstalk" of bosoms. Next will come your belly. Eventually your new Dolly-esque breasts will be dwarfed by your Budda-esque belly. In the end, the fat could accumulate on your butt, your thighs, your face, basically everywhere that's covered with skin.

There's not much I can say about weight gain except it's going to happen. It's an important part of pregnancy and it's a crucial factor in having a healthy baby. Some women seem to gain the most weight with their first kid. When pregnant with their second, it was harder to pack on the pounds while chasing after a toddler. Others found that they gained more with their second child. After the first was born, their cupboards were stocked with tempting toddler goodies, and of course, they had to finish off their child's plate of food. There seems to be no rhyme or reason to pregnancy weight gain except that it's as certain as death, taxes, and rain at an outdoor wedding.

A New Wardrobe

Yeah! You're pregnant! Not only are you going to be blessed with God's greatest creation, but you get to buy new clothes as well! I bet you can't wait; I know I couldn't.

The first time I had trouble buttoning my pants, I rushed down to my local maternity boutique. My mom met me so we could bond—sort of the women's equivalent of a father and son ice fishing trip. It was such fun to try on pregnancy clothes. I'd pull all that extra tummy material out to see how I'd look in the months to come, and laugh at the reflection. Yeah, like I'm really gonna get *that* big! I wore each outfit with pride, just like I did with my first Brownie uniform. For both then and now, I was a member of a very exclusive club.

But then it happened. The reflection that I laughed at just a few months before soon became a reality. And the clothes that brought a smile to my face brought tears to my eyes. For it wasn't long before those tent-like outfits didn't fit my ever-expanding tent-like frame.

I have a few words of wisdom to pass on to you in hopes of making your clothing experiences a little more enjoyable.

1. There are products you can purchase to widen the waistband of your pants, allowing you to fit into your regular clothes for several more weeks. You can buy them at maternity stores and on the Internet; but if you can't find them, just loop a rubber band around your top pant button, put it through the button hole, then back around the button. Your pants should stay up just fine without having to be fully buttoned. This trick will also work for your husband after he eats that foot-long sub.

2. Think disposable. Unless you have money to burn, I suggest going down to your local discount store and loading up on less expensive clothes. The outfits at your specialty maternity shops are cute, but expensive. I found this to be a case where quantity is better than quality.

3. When it comes to shoes, think slip-ons. It will get to the point where it'll become a struggle to tie up your shoelaces. I lived in a pair of clogs. With clogs, you just slip them on and start your day. Since I hadn't worn a pair since junior high, it did take some time to get used to them; but in the end, it was like riding a bike.

4. Borrow anything you can, but keep in mind that pregnancy clothes are hard to take care of. I steered away from borrowing anything nice because I knew that I probably couldn't return it in the same condition. I was clumsy and spilled a lot. I would sit on things since looking down required so much effort. And needless to say, I stretched the clothes out like Silly Putty.

5. Don't buy everything at once. Get a few pieces each month so that you'll always have something new to wear. This way you tend not to get so sick of your wardrobe than if you bought everything all at one time. You also get to treat yourself to something that's going to make you feel good about yourself. Though at the end, don't expect miracles. By then, the only thing that's going to make you feel good about yourself is not ripping a seam.

6. Look for prepackaged pregnancy sets like Belly Basics. They're five separate color-coordinated pieces that mix and match to create different outfits. They're sort of like Garanimals for the expecting. Try *www.babystyle.com* or maternity wear shops.

The amount of clothes you'll need will depend on your lifestyle. Do you work in an office that requires you to wear a suit? Do you go out a lot and need fancy clothes for dinner and the theater? You'll also need more clothing if you live in an area with distinct seasons. Living in L.A. and working at a job where overalls were considered elegant attire, I kept my new wardrobe at the minimum.

The Name Game

Although it's quite early in your pregnancy, it's hard to stop thinking about names. "Embryo" or "Fetus" is fine for now, but you'll need something more substantial later on.

One of the main reasons that I'm only going to have one child is that I can't go through the agony of choosing another name. It's such a monumental decision and I am such an indecisive person. I get brain freeze whenever I'm asked to choose between paper and plastic. I would have given anything if kids, like Cabbage Patch dolls, could come out with cute little names sewn onto their rear ends.

One obstacle that my husband and I had to overcome was that we are of different religions. In mine, we're supposed to name a child after a loved one who has passed away, and in my husband's, an offspring is named after someone still alive, namely . . . themselves. Don't get me wrong, I adore my in-laws but when I met them for the first time, I was amazed by how many children were named after their fathers. It was either "big" this or "little" that or "junior" or "the third." There were so many people who had the same name it was like going to George Foreman's family reunion.

So here we were, faced with the problem of not being able to name our child after someone dead or alive. I bought a book that listed some 15,000 names, and believe me, we considered each and every one of them. I guess the author had to do a lot of creative naming in order to get exactly 15,000 names. This book even contained the name "Happy," which I don't consider to be a name at all, except for those who whistle while they work.

At this point, we didn't know if our baby was a girl or boy so we discussed many names. If we found a name we liked, either it didn't sound good with our last name, or it reminded us of someone in our past that we would rather forget. There was one name he loved, but it was the same as my childhood swim teacher whom I feared because his second toe was bigger than his first. And every time I liked a name, it turned out to be the same as one of his ex-girlfriends.

After a couple dozen of my names were rejected, we stopped discussing names entirely and moved on to a much louder discussion.

But finally it happened. After months and months of agonizing debate, we had the name of our child (by then we knew the sex so there were 50 percent fewer choices to consider). Proud and excited, we announced the chosen name at the next family function. *Big mistake!* Rule number one of choosing a name for your child (and there is only one rule): Don't *ever* tell your family the name you decide upon until the child is born and the birth certificate is signed. I promise you that there will be someone in your family who will object to this name and will have no qualms about airing his or her true feelings. And even though you say it won't matter if everyone doesn't like the name you chose, it will.

So, we went back to the drawing board. Again, the headaches and the indecision. I liked cute spunky names; my husband preferred old-fashioned ones. It was a hard compromise. The pressure was getting to us, especially because, by then, I was deep in my eighth month.

It wasn't until we went away for the weekend for our anniversary that a name came to us. We stayed at a quaint little bed-and-breakfast, which had a cat as a mascot. My husband suggested that we name our child after the cat and, like a miracle, I agreed. It wasn't until a week or so later that Oprah said that this name was the second most common children's name. Because of this, I lost interest in it, but didn't have the strength to go back to that drawing board again. So we kept the name. My husband loves it. The family loves it. Me, I'm not so sure. To this day, I'm tempted to change it again. But then, I'm still regretting my decision to go with plastic instead of paper.

Your Newfound Celebrity

Being pregnant is similar to being a celebrity. Once someone finds out that you're expecting, it's as if you've been given a guest shot on *Will & Grace*. People will start to treat you differently. You'll get lots of attention. You'll be given the better chair. Every conversation will focus around you.

As your pregnancy progresses, it's as if your acting career has progressed as well. You're now getting film roles. You'll get seated quickly in crowded restaurants. People will give you their place in line. Someone will help you load your groceries into your car. And best of all, you can now take the good parking spots away from others without them getting upset. Once other drivers notice who you are, they'll be honored to give their spaces away.

I know that this newfound fame sounds great, and it is for a while. But soon, your fame, along with your belly, will grow bigger and bigger and bigger. You're now the star of Spielberg movies. People will stop and stare at you everywhere you go. They'll turn their heads and point like you're a car wreck on the side of the road. They'll try not to, but they won't be able to help themselves. After all, they're only human. And you, my friend, are larger than life.

You may find all this attention bothersome. Many superstars find it difficult as well. They become reclusive or wear disguises when they go out. But you have one major advantage over them. Your fame is fleeting and will end in a day. For the moment that you deliver your baby, you'll become a "pregnancy has-been." You'll go from Jennifer Aniston to Jennifer Grey in 10 centimeters. And from that moment on, you will take your place in the background while your baby becomes the new superstar. So, enjoy it while you can before the red carpet is pulled out from underneath you.

Drooling

I bet you think I made a mistake. What does drooling have to do with pregnancy? "Oh," you say, "I bet she meant to do a segment on drooling in an upcoming baby book. Yes, that must be it. How embarrassing for her." Then you let out a little chuckle. But, unfortunately, the chuckle's on you, because drooling is yet another curve in the roller coaster ride of pregnancy.

For some reason, expectant women produce a lot more saliva. They produce a lot more fluids in general like blood and pee. But for now, let's concentrate on spit. From what I remember from my high school physiology class, saliva is the first step in digestion. It seems that saliva contains an enzyme that starts to break down food as soon as it's in your mouth, making it easier to be digested when it arrives in your stomach. (Mr. Simcox really was an excellent teacher.) Now, as we've already learned from the segment on gas, your digestive system slows down in order to squeeze every nutrient from your food, so it makes sense that your body produces more saliva to help start off the process. And, if you're nauseated, your mouth seems to fill up with even more spit.

Although basically gross, there really isn't anything very troublesome about extra saliva. You might wake up on a soggy pillow. You may tend to spit your "P"s more when you

❝ I carried a cup around with me to spit into, but eventually, I got lazy and just spit into the carpet. I was so nauseous all the time I didn't really care. But then my two-year-old started copying me and would spit all over the house. ❞
—Kathleen

talk. My only advice is that you'll want to keep a tissue handy for any emergency drooling episodes. And, if you're practicing dental hygiene of some kind, stay close to the sink. Both brushing and flossing will produce an enormous amount of saliva and you'll need a nearby place to spit.

If you're suffering from drool big-time, make sure to brush your teeth before you get dressed in the morning. Spit plus toothpaste is a dangerous drooling combination and can create noticeable white streaks on fashionable office attire. If you're forced to brush after dressing, safety-pin a towel on yourself like a bib.

But generally speaking, a mouthful of spit doesn't hurt, and that's the important thing.

My Bloody Nose

An interesting fact to spread at cocktail parties is that a pregnant woman has about 25 percent more blood than a nonpregnant one. At first I thought this must be the reason for all my bloody noses. It made sense that with all this new blood coursing through my veins, something was going to blow— sort of like an old garden hose hooked up to a high-pressure valve. Undoubtedly, there are going to be a few cracks here and there. I thought nosebleeds were analogous to some of those cracks.

But the truth is that nosebleeds are caused by other things than all your extra blood. One thing is that those ever-abundant pregnancy hormones are turning your mucous membranes into mush, thus making them easier to break. Another reason is that your nasal tissues tend to dry out. I know this seems rather odd, since your body is retaining enough water to put out a small brushfire, but it's true.

I was never one to get nosebleeds in the past. I always

> **"** My nose would bleed whenever I'd blow it. I'd put the bloody tissues in the trash, and I know this sounds gross, but my dog would take them out and chew them up. There was something about the blood that he liked. **"**
>
> —Leslie

wanted them as a kid. They looked so dramatic, they got lots of attention, and they always warranted a trip to the nurse's office. The only thing I ever got were freckles, which got me nothing but teased.

But be warned, because even though the nosebleed is a pretty painless event there are a few things that you should be aware of:

1. A nosebleed can happen without any warning. It requires no sneezing, blowing, or picking of the nasal cavity whatsoever.
2. A nosebleed can do a great deal of damage to your wardrobe. I suggest that you stock up on a good stain remover for your laundry.
3. Wear a lot of earth tones, such as dark reds and browns, even if you're not an "autumn" complexion. It may not complement your skin tone, but at least people won't notice the spots of dried blood on your shirt.

You may not be able to stop nosebleeds entirely, but there are a few things you can do to lessen their frequency:

1. Rub a small dab of Vaseline around the inside of your nostrils.
2. Use a saline spray like Ocean Mist. It'll keep things wet up there.

3. Move to a tropical paradise. The humidity will do wonders for your nose as well as your complexion. If that's not possible, buy a humidifier.

Beware of Your Nipples

Let's get the human anatomy lesson over with. Your nipples are actually made up of two parts. The nipple itself is the raised part in the center that's made up of dense skin, and the round mass of pigmented skin that encircles it is called the areola (a pretty name to consider if you're having a girl). That said, both of these parts of your anatomy are in for a rocky ride over these next several months. Let me take you through their incredible journey.

First off, your areolae will change colors. Now, don't freak. I'm not talking about neon green or fuchsia. But your nipples will probably darken, especially if you had lighter-hued ones to begin with. I'm no areola expert, but it seems to me that their color is analogous to a good piece of steak. It can be anywhere from a pinkish "rare" to a charbroiled shade of "well done." And, as your baby cooks in your oven, so do your areolae.

Soon you'll notice that your areolae will start to grow. My areolae, which started off being the size of a quarter, grew to about a buck fifty. And every time I looked at them, they seemed to be getting even bigger. Eventually it seemed like they were taking over my entire body—like mold invading a piece of bread. I've heard the reason for areolae to grow and darken is to make them easier for your baby to find when it's trying to nurse. My kid would have to had the aim of a blind man to miss these targets.

Not only will the size of your areolae change, so will their texture. What used to be smooth and silky, will become hard and lumpy. These lumps are actually sweat glands that, for some unknown reason, decide to make an unwelcome appearance. Not only will your sweat glands rise and shine, so will your Montgomery glands. These glands, that are located around the rim of your areolae, will become lumpy as well. Although the lumps may not be too attractive, they will serve a purpose later on. They'll toughen up your nipples, getting them ready for breastfeeding. Babies may not have teeth, but their gums are strong and they're not afraid to use them.

In addition to the lumps provided by nature, you'll need to toughen up your areolae yourself. About the seventh month, while in the shower, you should start to rub them gently with a washcloth for about five or ten seconds. Afterwards, apply some moisturizer to them. Soon, your nipples will be so tough you can use them to scrub away baked-on lasagna. If you experience any contractions while rubbing your nipples, stop. In rare cases, even minor stimulation can cause contractions.

Now let's turn our attention to your nipples. Somewhere around the fourth month and continuing until delivery, your nipples may leak a yellow substance, colostrum, which is the precursor to breast milk. It's thick like wood glue but without the durable holding power. Colostrum is breast milk without the high fat content. If your nipples do indeed leak, it'll only be a drop or two. You may not even notice the drops, just some dry white flakes around your nipples after you've taken off your bra.

If leaking colostrum through your nipples isn't enough to make you say, "Gross!" maybe this will. Sometime, along with the colostrum, you may also leak blood. It's true. You see, the vessels inside your nipples are engorged with all your new pregnancy blood, and some of it may leak out from time to time as well. Yes, between your bloody nose, bloody gums, occasional spotting, and bloody nipples, you could donate to the blood bank without being hooked up to an IV.

The last nipple note is that as your breasts prepare to start feeding your child, your nipples will start to stick out more and become harder. They can get so big and pointy that it may surprise you. You may want to run out and buy a cone bra like the one Madonna used to wear. Mine felt so hard that I swore I could get work as an engraver.

But, when all is said and done, I have some good news for you. After you deliver (or stop breastfeeding if you chose to do so), your nipples and areolae will revert back to almost their prepregnancy size (at least mine did). Mine are a bit darker than they were, but at least they're smooth once again. My days of doing dishes without an S.O.S. pad are over.

Chapter Four

The Fourth Month

*H*ooray for you! You've made it through the first trimester! This is quite an accomplishment for several reasons. First, you're one-third of the way there! This is a big *X* to mark off on your pregnancy calendar. Second, you should be noticing that your morning sickness will probably start to fade. And last, but definitely not least, if you made it this far, there is a much greater chance that your baby will go to full term. Statistically speaking, if you get through the first trimester, you have over a 90 percent chance of going the distance.

I know for my husband and me, this was a great thing. After experiencing one miscarriage firsthand, we could breathe a little bit deeper now, and start to count on this one. Once again, I was as happy as I could have been (considering my condition).

You may have heard the same things that I did about the second trimester. I was told that it was the best trimester of them all. Crossing this trimester bridge meant that now I was going to be filled with energy like never before. The worst part was behind me and I would finally understand the magic of pregnancy!

"Great!" I thought. Finally, I was going to *like* being pregnant. I would be like the rest of womankind, experiencing the joy that growing a life force inside my belly could bring. I was now a part of the human evolution chain and I was going to carry that chain around my neck with pride! Little did I know that chain would become an anchor that I'd have to lug around with me for two more trimesters.

As it turned out, I did enjoy the second trimester more than the other two but for a different reason. It was the first time that I could greet the day without my head in a toilet bowl. My headaches and sore breasts were gone and I had overcome the withdrawal symptoms for that morning cup of Joe. Yes, by and large, I guess I was pretty amazed with what the second trimester would bring: a whole new list of ailments that I would have to endure.

Hyperemesis

I hate even mentioning the word "hyperemesis." First of all, most of you won't know what it means, and second of all, if you do, you know it's a very bad thing. Hyperemesis means severe morning sickness and it doesn't always go away after the first trimester.

There seem to be three levels of morning sickness. The first level is when you can cure it by eating a cracker. The second is when you feel nauseated and miserable all day long. You can still go to work, but you'll probably be spending some of your time lying facedown on the floor. The third, and by far the worst kind of morning sickness, is called hyperemesis.

With hyperemesis, you tend to lose a lot of weight

because you can't keep anything down. You're also spending a great deal of time gagging and throwing up. You can be in the middle of a sentence and then "kerblewie." And worst of all, there's a chance (albeit slim) that hyperemesis can last the duration of your pregnancy.

If you have hyperemesis, you can try any of the things suggested for morning sickness (see Morning, Noon, and Night Sickness on page 10). In addition, it's crucial to drink fluids so you won't become dehydrated. This is very important because you'll no doubt be vomiting a lot throughout the day. Water is best but sports drinks, ginger ale, and broth are acceptable, too. Basically anything that you can pour into a cup will do. Watch out for signs of dehydration like dizziness, disorientation, and dark yellow pee. If you experience any (or all) of these symptoms, call your doctor. Another way to deal with hyperemesis is to get a mute button on your telephone at the office. This way, you can conduct international conference calls and still gag from time to time without anyone being the wiser.

Hyperemesis can also make you sensitive to light, sound, and touch. Some people prefer to lie down in a dark quiet room. My neighbor Hallie did. She put herself on self-inflicted bed rest and would spend all day in her own personal hell. She did have an occasional visitor, but it had to be understood beforehand that if she threw up in midsentence, it must be ignored.

In addition to the basic remedies to morning sickness, your doctor can prescribe some drugs. Hallie took a new drug called Zofran. It was developed to lessen the nausea in cancer patients who were going through chemotherapy. These pills are very expensive, about $35 each, and you need to take three a day. If you have good insurance, it might cover it, but you'd be smart to check first. If not, there are several other medications to choose from, and most of these should be covered.

Although these drugs are no cure-all, they will make you well enough to keep some food down. Hallie ended up gaining 70 pounds during her pregnancy after she started taking Zofran! She now wishes she could get a small bout of hyperemesis to help her lose some of the baby weight.

Sex During the Second Trimester

Every time I came home from my doctor's appointment during the second trimester, my husband would ask if we got the okay to have sex again. Remember, we had been told to have complete pelvic rest during the first trimester. After my fourteenth-week appointment, I came home and gave my husband the good news. We had been given the green light. My husband looked at me like a released prisoner, grabbed me, and planted a kiss on me that made my toes curl. Even though it had been some time since we had been together, I distinctly noticed a difference in sex when I was pregnant. Things happened faster and with more intensity. Pregnancy sex is like regular sex on Miracle-Gro.

One of the reasons that it was so good is that the morning sickness had finally run its course. Like a woman who had a near-death experience, I wanted to live each day (or night) to its fullest. After morning sickness, everything was better, not just sex. Food tasted sweeter; air smelled cleaner; whites looked whiter. Everyday I was Julie Andrews spinning atop the mountain in *The Sound of Music*.

Another reason that sex is so much better is all the extra blood coursing though your veins (as well as other parts of your anatomy), which makes everything more sensitive. Yes, the reason you have bloody gums, noses, and nipples is the same reason you're having so much fun doing the nasty.

On top of that, this additional blood is full of additional hormones. Some of these must be the exact same hormones that sixteen-year-old boys have because, like them, all you can think about is sex. Now I know why I've never seen a teenage boy with his shirt tucked in.

I have so much respect for Mother Nature (and all mothers now that I'm one of them), but this is the first time I didn't understand her motives. Why should a woman want sex so much at a time when she is assured she can't conceive? Maybe Mother Nature is just being kind. She's giving you this final sexual hurrah because she knows that after the baby is born, it's going to be the last thing on your mind.

I was lucky. Not only did I enjoy having pregnancy sex, but my husband is one of those men who actually finds expectant women sexy. I don't understand how my bulging rotund stature turned him on, but I was flattered. I hear a lot of men have a difficult time making love to their pregnant wives, not because of their figure, because of the figure growing inside them. Even though the doctor says that sex won't hurt the baby, some men are afraid that it will. There's also some psychological stuff going on about you becoming a mother, and whenever the thought of a mother pops up in your husband's mind during sex, it's always a cause of concern.

Granted, there are some women who don't experience this increased sex drive. Some find that the increased sensitivity makes touch uncomfortable. Some are emotionally confused about their new role as mother versus their old role as wife. Some are having severe mood swings. If this is happening to you, relax. It's temporary. But I do send you my condolences. If it had happened to me, this book would have been titled *Pregnancy Really Sucks*.

The Ultrasound

One of the bonuses of pregnancy, along with the thick hair and long, vitamin-induced fingernails, are the ultrasounds. I say "ultrasounds" because you may have several of them. If you've had a miscarriage before, or are not sure how far along you are, you'll get a chance to see your kid very early in the pregnancy. Nothing will assure you that everything's okay in there like having a medical expert take a look and tell you it is.

We had our first ultrasound at seven weeks. It was so amazing to peer into my belly and see my child. Actually, it wasn't much of a child. It was more like a vibrating grain of rice. But it was our grain of rice and it was beautiful. We got our souvenir photo printout and proudly showed off our precious Uncle Ben to everyone who came within a ten-foot radius.

We had our next ultrasound at nineteen weeks (you may have one earlier or later depending on your doctor's advice). I admit that I was irrationally nervous. There was part of me that was expecting to see that fetal pig inside my uterus. So, you can imagine my joy and elation to see an actual human child on the ultrasound screen. What a miracle it was to witness the transformation from rice grain to baby in only eleven

> **"** My husband and I were watching the ultrasound and we saw a long protrusion coming from our baby's thigh. My husband raised his fist triumphantly and shouted 'That's my boy!' The doctor explained that he was looking at the umbilical cord. **"**
>
> —Kate

weeks. This grain now had ten fingers and ten toes and not a trace of a curly tail anywhere.

The doctor gave us a tour of our unborn child, explaining that this blob was the arm and that blob was the foot. We "oohed" and "aahed" and pretended to see what he was pointing out. Seeing your child with ultrasound technology is like trying to understand modern art.

The doctor also gave our child its first physical exam. He studied its internal organs, digestive system, brain development, and bone density. He did everything but have the fetus bend over and cough. We were told how much junior weighed and how tall junior was. And then we were even given the option of knowing if junior was a boy or a girl.

My husband and I had discussed this option in great length beforehand. He wanted to wait until our child was born to find out the sex. He said that it'd be such a great surprise. I thought it'd be surprising enough to see a human spring from my innards. I wanted to know the sex as soon as possible. I told him that if we knew, we could bond with it better. We could pick out a name and know what color to paint the room. We could start buying cute little baby clothes that are so tiny they could be worn as a brooch. But the truth is, the real reason I wanted to know is that I'm just an incredibly impatient person.

I made a deal with my husband that if we found out the sex *this* time, we would wait to find it out with our next child. This sounded like a fair deal to him so he agreed. Sucker. (Like there would ever be a next time!)

We told the doctor that we wanted to know the sex and the search was on. He found the appropriate area and then showed us what we were looking for. He announced that our baby had three dots! This confused us a bit. I figured we'd either see something sticking out or going in. Nowhere in my sex education classes had we discussed three dots.

The doctor explained that three dots meant that it was a girl. A girl! We were having a girl! My husband asked the doctor if he was sure, and the doctor told him that he was. But still my husband had his doubts, I can't say I blame him. I don't see how the existence of three dots translates to a girl either. I've seen plenty of naked women in locker rooms and I've never noticed any of them having three dots.

You, of course, will have your own ultrasound experience. You may very well have more ultrasounds than we had. Either way, I guarantee it will be one of the most memorable moments of your life. Yes, yes, yes, I know that this book is about how much pregnancy can suck, but I just had to throw in one morsel of glee. Besides, there are still a few things that I want to advise you about.

1. Make sure that you bring a blank VHS tape with you. Don't assume that the doctor's office has them on hand. Yes, I know that in all the movies and television shows, the doctor hands the teary-eyed couple a tape of the ultrasound. But in real life it's not automatic. We didn't have a blank tape on hand, but luckily, they had an extra one. We must have watched that tape twenty times that week, and I would have been quite upset if we didn't have it.

2. Bear in mind that body parts can look awfully confusing on an ultrasound monitor. Although your technician can identify every nook and cranny of your in utero baby, don't get worried if you see extra or missing body parts.

3. Don't think your kid will look anything like the image that appears on the screen. I'm sure in the not-too-distant future, an ultrasound will have the quality of a digital camera, but for now, it's more like an x-ray that shows the skeletal being inside of you. Even though I loved my "skeletoid" as much as anyone could, I admit that she was butt ugly.

Hollow eye sockets, enormous head, and a nose as big as a "before" picture of an extreme rhinoplasty. This kid was destined to go to the prom with her cousin.

I'm Scared!

By now, or maybe sometime before now, the fear has set in. You're going to have a baby! The words that brought such joy to your life are causing such pains in your chest. Even though having a child may be what you've always wanted, the actual thought of it can be terrifying.

One of my big fears was that I was going to be a terrible mom. I mean, I'd never actually been one before, so how would I know how I'd do? I can't even keep a houseplant alive for more than a couple of weeks. The only practical experience I had at childrearing was the babysitting I did as a teenager. And even then, I wasn't very good at it. I once dropped my little cousin Alexis headfirst on a hardwood floor. Was I insane to believe that I could take care of a child?

Another one of my worries was that I started the procreation process too late. I was constantly calculating how old I would be when my kid went to kindergarten or drove a car. Man, I was going to be old! I wondered who was going to be in a walker first, her or me?

I'm sure that you have fears of your own about being pregnant. A common worry is that you may have caused harm to your unborn child. Did that cold medicine you took before you knew you were pregnant harm the embryo? Or you may be worried that your husband will never want to make love to you after he watches the baby being born. How could he want to touch you after seeing so many bodily fluids come out at one time? Or what about the fear of not being able to get your body back in shape? Or losing touch with your girlfriends? I bet you lost some friends when they had kids. All they ever wanted to talk about was their kids' poop.

I think, by far, the most common fear is that of giving up your life, and it's a fear that's very well founded. You've already had to give up many of your favorite things in order to get where you are now, and you know that there'll be plenty more sacrifices in store for you for years and years to come. In a few short months, you'll be giving up sleep, the luxury of going to the bathroom without an audience, to chew your food without interruptions, or to have one complete uninterrupted thought. You'll give up the indulgence of talking on the phone whenever you wish, of letting the cream rinse sit on your head for the required three minutes, and of having a clean house for more than a twenty-minute stretch. Sorry, once I got going, it was hard to stop myself.

But fret not. Like every good comparison shopper, I'll provide you with a list of pros and cons to get a better perspective on what's to come. Just remember, when one door closes, another one opens. And it's a good thing too, because sometimes, you're going to want to throw yourself right out of it.

What You're Giving Up	*What You're Getting*
Hourglass figure	Hourly feedings
Fancy restaurants	Fast-food restaurants
Bank CDs	Barney CDs
Loads of sex	Loads of laundry
Dirty movies	Dirty diapers
Island getaways	Disneyland getaways

What You're Giving Up	*What You're Getting*
Party all night	Up all night
Television	Teletubbies
Cocktail parties	Pin the Tail parties
Perky breasts	Leaky breasts
Honeymoon	*Goodnight Moon*
Happy life	Happy Meals

But, what it all boils down to is:

What You're Giving Up	*What You're Getting*
Your whole life	A brand-new life

And that alone makes it all worthwhile.

Vaginal Discharge

I know the term "vaginal discharge" sounds gross, but get used to it. You're naive if you think the only thing that's going to come out of there is a baby. Mucous plugs, bloody show, and the placenta are but a few of the coming attractions. But the vaginal discharge that I'm referring to now is called *leukorrhea*.

Somewhere around the fourth month, you'll notice that your underwear has a distinct spot on the crotch. This spot is white and creamy and looks like it should be applied around the eyes to reduce the appearance of fine lines and wrinkles.

Although there is no way to stop the flow of leukorrhea,

some women try anyway. Because of this, I want to warn you of two things that you should never do while pregnant:

1. Don't use tampons. Tampons prevent normal bacteria from escaping through your vagina, which could lead to infection. Here you are, abstaining from your favorite things like alcohol, cigarettes, and chocolate in order to have a healthy child. You'd hate to ruin it all by one superabsorbent wand.

2. Don't douche. I'm not quite sure why women douche in the first place. I always heard a vagina is like a self-cleaning oven, but, to each her own. Just don't do it while you're pregnant.

Although leukorrhea is not at all painful or uncomfortable, there is one problem. It stains. You can bleach your tidy whities till you're blue in the face, but they'll never be tidy again. If they could turn this discharge into exterior house paint, they'd have a substance that could survive years of harsh winters without cracking or fading. Although you can't stop the flow from a comin', you can prepare for it somewhat.

The best way to deal with leukorrhea is to load up on disposable underwear. I suggest you take a ride down to your local discount store and stock up on Hanes. They're cheap, cotton, and oh-so-darn cute. After your belly gets too big though, get the cheap maternity underwear. If you like, you can buy the high-rise kind that covers your whole belly. Personally, I didn't like them. Not only didn't I like the chuckles I'd get from my husband (they are rather comical looking), but I found that wearing anything on my belly was irritating.

If the thought of cheap disposable undies puts your tush

in an uproar, they do sell more expensive maternity bikinis that are cut lower in front. They also sell maternity thongs, although, if you prefer thongs, your nonpregnancy ones should fit you for your entire pregnancy without much of a problem. But if money's no issue, go ahead and buy the pricey, low-cut, sexy maternity undies. They'll probably make you feel a bit more attractive, which would be a good thing about now. But protect your investment. You can either have your panties Teflon-coated, or load up on panty shields. I know that wearing panty shields day in and day out for nine months may be a bit expensive, but who said having a kid would be cheap? There are all kinds of hidden costs in the child-rearing biz, and panty shields are just one of them.

If you aren't able to wear your prepregnancy underwear, hide them away. There may be times that seeing those lacy numbers will remind you of your old self and bring tears to your eyes. You're feeling weepy most days anyway. If you think a Hallmark commercial is difficult to watch, just wait till you see what an old pair of your sexy lace bikinis do to you.

Toilet Troubles

Yup, face it, you have toilet troubles. You try and try, but you just can't poop. You try so hard that you're afraid you're going to push the baby out. Don't laugh, you know you've thought about it. You may believe that all this pushing will be good practice for labor, but the only thing it's good for is causing hemorrhoids.

First of all, I'm going to explain to you why you're constipated. It won't help you go to the bathroom, but it will help you understand what's going on with the being you used to call your body. The number one reason for your number two

> **"**I was so constipated that my doctor told me to give myself an enema. I got one and did it on the living room floor. When I was stood up I looked out the window and noticed some neighbors watching me from across the alley.**"**
>
> —Iliana

problem is that your baby is growing. Because of this, the light of your life is pressing into your bowels. It's sort of like stepping on a running garden hose. When you do this, less water will come out. Even if you turn on the water pressure (like when you push hard), it still doesn't open up the hose, it just causes it to leak (i.e., a hemorrhoid).

The second reason for all this constipation is all those darned hormones again. Progesterone, a critical hormone for the growth of the baby, causes your digestive system to become sluggish. Because of this, things tend to get backed up a bit. But how can you be so mad at a hormone that's keeping your baby warm, safe, and snug?

The third and final reason for all this blockage are those evil prenatal vitamins. If you read the ingredients, you'll find that they contain a large dose of iron. It must be real iron since it turns your poop into steel.

Now that you understand why you can't go, doesn't it make it all better? No? Okay, then here are some things that you can do when the going gets tough:

1. Keep hydrated.
2. Take a stool softener. In fact, get a truck full. You're going to find that stool softeners are going to be your best friend even after the baby is born too (but we'll get to that later).

3. Take a laxative like Senekot or Milk of Magnesia. Laxatives may have some side effects, but so does severe constipation. If all else fails, get your doctor's approval and try it.

4. Take a fiber supplement.

5. Cross your fingers that you're anemic. When you're anemic, you'll be given iron pills. Yes, I know that I said that iron clogs you up, but iron pills for anemia contain a wonderful ingredient that turns your poop into farina.

6. If you're not anemic, ask you doctor if you can switch to a low-iron prenatal vitamin.

7. Use a footstool when it's time to push. (A stool for your stool, so to speak.)

Constipation is something that tends to stick with you throughout your pregnancy. I know it sounds rough to endure for so long, but face it, some aspects of pregnancy are pretty crappy.

Bloody Gums

Making a baby is a team effort for your entire body. Your heart has to beat-faster. Your digestion has to slow down. But one of the most beat-up parts of your anatomy is your gums. They, like the rest of you, are pretty swollen. They're tender and engorged and because of this, they tend to bleed easily.

I can't tell you how many times I brushed my teeth only to find that my toothbrush was red and my floss was full of blood. I would bite into an apple and it would become streaked like a tie-died shirt. I became a vampire's dream.

Luckily, this occasional bleeding doesn't hurt, doesn't keep you up nights, and doesn't require any expensive remedies.

In fact, there are no remedies. But because your gums are working overtime, it's important to take care of them. This means, of course, (cue scary music) going to the dentist!

It is important to see a dentist at least once while you're pregnant so you don't make this gum problem worse. I don't recommend that you go during your first trimester when you're nauseated. I already told you about that gag reflex that may cause you to throw up if anything goes into your back teeth. Yes, vomiting all over your dentist may make you feel better for the suffering she inflicted upon you during that root canal, but take a pass anyway. But make sure you tell your dentist that you're pregnant so she won't take x-rays or give you any drugs. This makes for a very short appointment, which I certainly didn't complain about. Yes, even *I* didn't complain about that.

Genetic Testing

When it comes to genetic testing, you can either choose door number one, or door number two. The first choice is called a CVS. It stands for a bunch of long multisyllabic words that I don't know how to spell. Your second choice is amniocentesis. Both tests are used to detect chromosomal disorders in your unborn child. They're usually given for two reasons. One reason is if the mother will be thirty-five years or older upon delivery since the prevalence of genetic disorders increases with age. If you are, you'll be given the flattering label of AMA (advanced maternal age). The second reason to have a genetic test is if you or the father has a history of chromosomal defects in the family. A common defect is Down syndrome, but there are a slew of other ones that are screened for as well. Keep in mind, you aren't forced to have either one of these tests. If you're certain that you wouldn't want to terminate your pregnancy if your child has a chromo-somal defect, then you can elect to decline this test entirely.

Before you have either the amnio or a CVS, you'll no doubt have some kind of genetic interview. This interview may be with your doctor or a genetic counselor. Either way, this counselor will go over your family history and ask you questions about the health of your siblings, your parents, and your grandparents. I found out that my husband's family has a history of heart disease, diabetes, and juvenile arthritis. Combine that with my family's history of mental illness and cancer, and it made us realize that we definitely needed better health coverage.

If you decide to go with a CVS, it's given early—some-where around your eleventh week of pregnancy. The test itself is no big deal. It sounds scary and is rather invasive, but from a patient's point of view, it's not much worse than a Pap smear. During your "smear," your doctor will actually remove a small piece of the placenta with the help of an ultrasound. Seeing your baby in ultrasound always helps you relax. They could pour hot lava up your nose and you really wouldn't care. This piece of placenta is then examined for any chromosomal problems and, of course, to determine the sex of the baby.

The good news about a CVS is that the results are given much earlier—within a couple of days—than with an amnio-centesis (or "amnio" as they say in the pregnancy biz). With an amnio, you may have to wait more than a week. I know that it's only a matter of a few extra days, but you'll find that you get more nervous with each day you don't get the results back. If you've ever taken an AIDS test, you'll understand what I mean.

The bad news about a CVS is that the test is much more dangerous. The chance of miscarriage with a CVS is one in 100, versus one in approximately 200 with an amnio. Your doctor may tell you different percentages, I'm just telling you what I've heard. Both tests are extremely accurate in terms of diagnosis.

Your second choice in genetic testing is called an amniocentesis. That's the one that I chose to have. You're probably more familiar with the procedure than with the CVS because it's been around for so much longer. The way an amnio works is simple. With the help of an ultrasound, the doctor uses a needle to draw out some amniotic fluid to analyze for chromosomal abnormalities. Unfortunately, the needle is the size of a barbeque skewer, and seeing your baby come inches from being a kabob is a bit scary. Because of this, I suggest that you turn your head.

I'll be honest. Although I thought the procedure would be incredibly painful, the truth was that it wasn't. But, even though it wasn't painful, it was quite uncomfortable. Once they got the needle inside there, the worst part was over. But it took a good deal of hard pushing to get the needle through the tough walls of my uterus. Isn't it ironic that the only muscle I never worked out is the strongest one of them all?

The whole thing takes but a minute and then it's over. There is some cramping for a little while afterward, but it isn't so bad. You're instructed to go home and rest for twenty-four hours. You must be driven home and the only heavy machinery you can operate is your telephone to order takeout. You must also be given a long back rub that night. Or at least that's what my husband thought (wink, wink).

Boy or Girl?

It's driving you crazy, isn't it? Come on, you can tell me. Even though you both agreed not to find out the sex of your child, you still want to know. You close your eyes and try to visualize what's inside. Do you feel sugar and spice and everything nice or snips and snails and puppy dog's tails?

I was pretty lucky. Even without the results of our amnio, I felt pretty sure that our child would be a girl. In my family, there really isn't any other choice. I'm one of two girls. I have six cousins—all girls. Now, my cousins who have children all have girls. We even had a cat when I was growing up that had a litter of kittens and, you guessed it, all girls. I know they say that it's the father who determines the sex of the child, but we women must have a Y chromosome fumigator buried deep in the lining of our uteruses.

You may have an idea as to what the sex of your child is. Maybe it came to you in a dream, or maybe it's just a gut feeling. But if you're clueless, there are plenty of old wives' tales that can help you out. These theories have been around for ages and have endured the test of time. I'd love to be able to tell you the history behind some of these wives' tales, but I've always hated history. Suffice to say that there have probably been some pregnant women who had one of these symptoms and then delivered either a boy or girl. Whatever the history, here's what the old wives have to say:

It's a Girl If You:	It's a Boy If You:
Carry high	Carry low
Crave sweets	Crave salty or sour food
Have a wide belly	Have a round belly
Hold weight in your tush	Hold weight in your stomach
Have strong morning sickness	Have little morning sickness

It's a Girl If You:	It's a Boy If You:
Have a large left breast	Have dark nipples
Your hair gets highlights	You have fast-growing leg hair
Your pee is light in color	Your pee is dark in color
Your baby has a fast heartbeat	Your baby has a slow heartbeat
Ring dangled over belly goes in circles	Ring dangled over belly sways from side to side
You won't eat the ends of bread	Your feet are cold

I know that some of these suggestions seem ridiculous, but who knows, maybe the old wives are right. Maybe they know something that neither you nor medical science is aware of, and they shouldn't be laughed at. I plan on being an old wife myself one day, and I hope that when I share a wee bit of knowledge I've learned through years of experience, I won't have people mocking me. So, let's raise a glass of milk in honor of these women of wisdom!

Chapter Five

The Fifth Month

So here you are, starting your fifth month! I bet you never thought you'd make it this far. A lot has happened by now for both you and your baby. You've grown five dress sizes; your baby's grown genitals. In fact, if your baby is a girl, this month she'll develop her uterus and start making her eggs. Just think, not only are you carrying around your baby, but all your future grandchildren as well. No wonder you're gaining so much weight.

I found the fifth month to be a pretty good one as far as pregnancy months go. It's sort of the eye of the reproduction hurricane. The aches and pains of the fifth month shouldn't be all that wretched. You can expect them to be somewhere between the pain of your past dry heaves and those of your future delivery. After five months you've had ample time to get used to experiencing some kind of daily discomfort and nuisance. But the best part of being in your fifth month is that your belly has grown large enough now so you definitely look pregnant, not just fat. No longer will your bank teller give you that "Wow, she's sure letting herself go" kind of look.

Of course, there'll be struggles. What would a good pregnancy month be without any struggles? There was many a day that I'd attempt to pick myself up by my bootstraps and keep on keeping on. Eh, who am I kidding? We both know that our feet are too swollen to get into our boots.

Maybe you need to take a break from reading this book. Maybe you don't want to hear about anymore pregnancy complaints. Maybe you wish you'd waited longer for science to perfect human cloning before you started to reproduce. So just relax. Before we dive into the fifth month, go to the kitchen and get yourself a bowl of ice cream. And while you're there, stick a cheek cell in the freezer in case technology is perfected in time for your next kid.

Pains Under Your Uterus

It seems that the entire weight of your growing fetus rests on two ligaments that are located underneath either side of your uterus. Before you had a "wombmate," these ligaments were about the diameter of your pinky. Now they're about the size of your husband's thumb. As the baby moves around inside you, it shifts its weight from side to side. This motion can cause one of those ligaments to spasm.

Ligament spasms are a fairly common complaint. They usually begin during the second trimester and can continue until delivery. They're probably the most common in the last month or two when your baby gets pretty heavy, putting more stress on your poor aching ligaments. In the scheme of horrendous pregnancy moments, ligament spasms don't rank as all that horrendous. I mention them merely to save you an embarrassing call to the doctor fearing that your baby is in peril yet again.

The first time I had a ligament spasm was when I was

walking my devil dog, the affectionate term I have for the beast I call my pet. As with most devil dogs, walking mine is not a leisurely activity, but rather a daily ritual that ends in heavy panting and drinking from the toilet (for me, not the dog).

Anyway, on one of these rituals when I was trying to stop the beast from attacking an elderly man in a walker, I had an incredible pain in my lower side. It came in an instant and left in about the same time. I thought maybe I had pulled something, but it was over so fast that I wasn't exactly sure what had happened. It wasn't but a few minutes later that I had another one, and then one more thrown in for good measure.

We raced home, which we would have done anyway with or without the pain, and I called my doctor in hysterics. Were these early labor pains? Was my baby becoming dislodged? My doctor assured me that these pains were normal. He explained ligament spasms to me in that cool, soothing tone that he reserves for hysterical first-time moms and patients in an insane asylum.

I had more "attacks" as the weeks went on. It seemed that these ligament pulls were clustered in groups of three or four at a time, and usually in the morning. They were also almost always on my right side. I guess my baby preferred one half over the other. Maybe they had opened up a Starbucks on that side and she needed her morning fix. They *are* popping up everywhere. I would get these pains from time to time, even more so during the last trimester.

About now, I would provide you with a list of things you can do to prevent ligament spasms. But there is no solution, at least nothing noted in a medical textbook. But I do have a piece of advice from one mother-to-be: golf. She said that there was something about the swing that reduced their occurrence. Maybe the swing would stretch her ligaments. Or maybe it would just relax her. Either way, if you get a lot of ligament spasms, maybe you should get your fanny to the fairway.

In terms of treating the pain of ligament spasms, there's not much you can do. By the time you could put a warm compress on it, it'd be over. They're yet another thing that you have to endure in order to become a mother. You should be keeping an ongoing list of things like this and show them to your child before each Mother's Day. Sure, this won't cure the spasm, but it may assure you a nice gift come each May.

Your Cheesy Belly

One night as I was lying in bed reading one of my dozens of pregnancy books, I had a horrifying experience. I put the book down and started to get out of bed, when suddenly, I caught a glimpse of my naked belly. As if the gross size of the thing wasn't horrifying enough, the shape of it had transformed from round to pointy. It was as if I were impregnated with a giant wedge of cheese.

I screamed for my husband who came racing into the bedroom as all good husbands with screaming wives should do. He took one look at my stomach and he too was taken aback. What the hell was growing inside me? As soon as I relaxed back onto the bed, my stomach returned to its normal round shape. I lifted myself up again, and again my tummy was pointy. It turned out that whenever I tightened up my stomach muscles, it looked as if our child put on a big foam cheese hat worn by a Green Bay Packer fan. This really ticked off my husband since he follows the Chiefs.

I had read in one of my books that your stomach muscles

start to separate as your belly expands, but I had no idea that it would go this far. My stomach muscles were so far apart they were almost on my back. It's very easy to tell if your muscles have separated yet by simply lying down on the floor and lifting your head up. If you look at your tummy and suddenly get a hankering for a hunk of Gouda, you too have started the morphing process.

This oddity can be quite entertaining. I showed off my cheese-child at the office Christmas party and was the hit of the evening. Maybe it was because I was a fat pregnant lady lying down on the floor with my shirt lifted up for the world to see, but either way, I was quite the hit.

After another month or two, you won't notice your cheese stomach anymore. Not because your stomach muscles have mysteriously joined together again (I'm still waiting for mine to go back), but because your belly will get so big that the only way to get up from your back will be to roll over onto one side.

I wish I could say that after your baby is born, your stomach muscles will line up again to where they were before, but the truth is, they don't. The only way to get those suckers back together again is situps and crunches.

I do have a secret to let you in on. You're probably going to think that I'm lying, but I swear it's true. I know of one doctor who will suture your abdominal muscles together again after delivery (I'm not naming names, but you can look at the cover of this book for a hint). This mystery doctor will only do this if your muscles are really far apart and if you need a C-section. I'm not sure if he's a rare breed, but you can certainly ask your doctor if he'd be willing to do this too. I've never heard about this secret before. I'd heard that doctors would add an extra stitch while sewing up a tear to tighten up her vagina, but I wasn't aware of tummy work as well. I guess having a baby is as good excuse as any to have a little work done.

You're So Vein

You may have noticed something new about your body since you've become pregnant. Actually, I don't think there's one part of your body that's still the same. The latest change you may notice is that something strange is happening to your veins.

One of the most noticeable changes is that your skin has turned into a road map. New highways and byways are popping up everywhere with the greatest construction site being around your chest. All of these new roads are actually veins and arteries that are more noticeable because of your body's increase in blood volume. Although your newfound body atlas isn't physically painful, you may encounter some venous changes that can hurt.

Varicose veins are one of those changes. Varicose veins are much more likely to appear in expectant women than in men, which is yet another reason to resent your spouse. One of the main reasons for the appearance of varicose veins is that your baby is acting like a dam, blocking the blood flow from your lower body back up to your heart. Because of your dam baby (sorry to offend), your leg veins expand. Inside the veins (those that are going up your legs) are little valves that open and close to let the blood pass through. But, because your veins are now larger, the valves don't close all the way, which allows blood to pool and collect.

These pools can occur anywhere from your ankle up to your vulva. They can be anywhere from the size of a raisin to that of a pear. And the pain that comes with them varies from mildly uncomfortable to major "owie." Varicose veins are usually hereditary, so a good way to tell if you're a candidate for getting them is to check out your mom's gams.

Another place to get a varicose vein (and I hope you're sitting on a soft pillow for this pronouncement) is your rectum. When you get a varicose vein there, it's actually called a hemorrhoid and we'll be discussing them later on in the book.

If you're at risk for varicose veins, there are some things you can do to prevent them:

- Wear support hose.
- Don't wear tight clothing.
- Take a long walk.
- Don't lift anything heavier than a fifteen-pound watermelon.
- And most important, don't sit too long or stand too long. When you're pregnant, you must be in constant motion like a shark.

Although most varicose veins will go away after the dam bursts (your baby is born), yours may be a bit more stubborn. If yours don't go away, there are several medical procedures, from laser to liposuction, to get rid of them. But, unless your varicose vein is extremely painful or just plain nasty looking like one that's on your vulva, wait until all of your kids are

❝ I was so veiny, it looked like you could see right through me. My daughter, who was in first grade at the time, brought me to class for show and tell when they were studying the human body. ❞

—Jody

born before you have them removed. It'd be like getting a breast lift after each child stops nursing.

The last vein change you may notice is spider veins. Unlike regular spider veins, the ones that occur when you're pregnant are caused by . . . you guessed it . . . hormones. Spider veins are dilated blood vessels that mostly appear in your legs. Although they're not very attractive, it won't be long before they won't bother you anymore. Not because they'll go away, but because your belly will become so enormous, that you won't even be able to see them (or anything else south of your belly button for that matter).

Although most of my newfound arachnid skin friends vanished after I delivered, some have stuck around (if this happens you can see a dermatologist). I know that a lot of women are really bothered by spider veins. Lucky for me, I have so many other worse conditions on my body, that they're the least of my concerns.

Who Asked You?

This just in: The Surgeon General has determined that people around a pregnant lady will become total idiots. I'm not sure why it happens, but you're going to find that strangers will no doubt tell you cruel things about your pregnancy. Things will sputter from their lips that will shock you beyond belief. And most surprising of all, they'll say it with a smile.

My first encounter with this amazing behavior was when I got into an elevator of an office building. There was one other woman inside who smiled and told me that I looked like I was about five months along. I told her she was exactly right and asked how she knew. She then said with the casualness of telling me the time, "Oh, that's how far along my neighbor was when she had her miscarriage." I was stunned but smiled stupidly and said "Oh, really?" Just then the doors opened, she said goodbye and left. I was in shock. How can a person just say a thing like that?

I'm not quite sure why it happens. Maybe people are born without a heart. Maybe they're born without a brain. Maybe the world is flooded with scarecrows and tin men and we don't even know it. I truly don't believe that people tell you these things to hurt you. I think they feel as if they're doing you some favor, like a public service announcement.

Everywhere you go, you'll be showered with unwanted information. So-called obstetricians and old wives will surround you at every turn. They'll be at checkout lines, gas stations, drug stores, and office parties, dispensing horror stories and free advice. Even your close friends and family members will have somehow gotten a medical license while you weren't looking and will freely share their newfound knowledge with you.

They'll drop in while you're cleaning and order you to stop. "Don't you know that polishing silver will damage your baby?" They'll watch you unpack groceries and scream, "Don't reach so high, you'll wrap the umbilical cord around the baby's neck!"

I'm not telling you this to scare you . . . but be afraid anyway. Be *very* afraid. For it will happen. The reason I'm telling you this is for one purpose only. So that maybe, when it happens to you, you won't spend so much time being as shocked as I was, and can respond to these fools with a witty comeback. I didn't do this. I just stood there like a jerk, sometimes even thanking them for their advice. It was only after they left that I thought of some brilliant retort.

Dear Abby would probably tell you to be polite to these dweebs. Me, no way. I feel it's your public duty to berate, belittle, and insult these stupid heads so they won't continue their damaging behavior. It's the kind thing to do. The only person that you should be taking advice from when you're pregnant is your doctor (and me, of course, but that goes without saying). That's my public service announcement, so there!

Third Nipples and Other Gross Things

For some women, like my cousin Amy, pregnancy can enhance the quality of your skin. Amy's skin glowed with such radiance that you couldn't look directly at her except through a pinhole in a piece of cardboard. Amy never wanted her pregnancy to end because she knew that, even though she would gain an offspring, she would lose that glow.

For me, pregnancy had the opposite effect. My skin was sallow and acne ridden. It would have been even more frustrating if I had had good skin to begin with, but it's usually pretty sallow and acne ridden. None the less, strange things began to happen during my second trimester that made it even worse.

By far the strangest thing was that I grew a third nipple. Yes, a third nipple. Freaky, huh? Before I conceived I had a slight discoloration a few inches under my right breast. It was small, about half the size of an M&M (regular, not peanut). But by the time I was in my fifth month, it got larger and darker, and by the time I delivered, it grew a bump in the center of it. I imagine that, with some effort, I could have gotten that thing to lactate.

I actually consider myself lucky that I only had one extra nipple. My doctor told me that there are two unseen nipple lines that go from your nipples down to your groin. A pregnant woman can actually have multiple nipples that, like mine, can get bigger during pregnancy.

In addition to the bonus nipple, I also found that my skin was developing broken capillaries. These little red dots started popping up everywhere. It was as if my entire body was being transformed into an astronomical map. Every day there'd be new constellations emerging on my chest, back, and face.

Even if you don't get a third nipple or broken capillaries, don't fret. There's a slew of other lovely skin problems that you may still encounter. One of my favorites is a skin tag. A skin tag is a small floppy growth of skin that grows around the areas of friction. Some ideal places are under the arm or in the folds of your neck skin, but anywhere skin rubs against skin could be a candidate. You can also get tags where your skin gets rubbed by clothing like your bra line. Skin tags don't do much. They don't hurt or itch, and if large enough, can probably be used to keep you warm on a cold winter's night.

One of the most common of all skin ailments is called PUPP. Although it sounds cute and cuddly, it couldn't be less so. PUPP stands for pruritic urticarial papules and plaques. That mumbo jumbo translates to a body riddled with itchy skin bumps. Fortunately, PUPP only happens in the last month or so of pregnancy. It starts around your belly button and spreads outward. The rash can be restricted to your belly, or travel to any other part of your anatomy except your face. PUPP is genetic and travels through your father's genes. Your mother will love this because she's no doubt been blamed for everything else that's gone wrong in your life.

There are two bits of good news about PUPPs. One is that there are things you can do to make your itching feel better. Cortisone cream is a good one. It should relieve the itching within a day or two. In really bad cases, your doctor can pre-scribe oral steroids. The other bit of good news is that you can only get PUPPs during your first pregnancy. That may not be too much of a comfort since you're convinced you'll never get yourself in this position again anyway. But you never know. If accidents never happened, I wouldn't be here and you'd be pretty upset that you spent money on a blank book.

But relax. Almost all skin problems go away when the baby is born. Both my third nipple and the astronomical map went away a few months after I gave birth. Of course I still have the sallow, acne-ridden complexion, but I guess having a baby is the only miracle I was going to get out of this pregnancy.

That's a Hormone of a Different Color

You may not know this—in fact, medical science is completely unaware—but pregnancy hormones are just like Easter egg dye coursing through your veins. And just like Easter egg dye, they make you change color. I've already told you about your areolae getting darker, but this increased pigmentation can happen anywhere on your body. Let's start on your head and work ourselves downward, shall we?

You may notice by now that your face has started to look darker than usual. Not an all-over bronze that makes you look as if you've just returned from the beach, but rather a patchy discoloration around your cheeks, nose, and forehead that makes you look as if you've just returned from the mines. If your skin is dark, your patches will be lighter toned. As with most skin problems, you should wear sunblock and a wide-brim hat. Or, just as nonpregnant women are advised, stay out of the sun entirely. Isn't it frustrating living on a planet where it's bad for you to go outside? Your local spa or facialist may suggest microdermabrasion, glycolic peels, or lightening gels to even out your complexion, but I'd steer clear of any of these treatments without an okay from your doctor. Usually just your regular makeup will be enough to cover up the blotches and smooth out your skin tone.

Moving south, look for a dark line to develop from your belly button down to your crotch. It's as if Mother Nature took out a black Sharpie and turned your belly into a doodle pad. This line used to be white and you probably never even noticed it before. But now that it's starting to darken, it's hard to miss. It was once called your *linea alba* when it was white, but now is referred to as your *linea nigra* (black line).

Next, be aware of your labia (that's a sentence I've never used before). It too will get darker. I know that you can't see anything below your waist anyway, but your husband still can and I feel he deserves to be warned.

Your hands and feet are also candidates for a color change. The palms of your hands and soles of your feet may become red and itchy. This is most common among white women, but every skin tone is vulnerable. In addition, your feet, and possibly even your legs, stand a chance of turning blue. It gets worse when it's cold outside, so make sure to keep your toes toasty. I assure you that your hands and feet will return to their normal skin tone after delivery. In the meantime, you can always run yourself up a flagpole on the Fourth of July.

In addition, it's not that uncommon for your body to develop moles. I admit to getting a few myself, but my neighbor's condition was far more severe. Vicky (name changed to protect the "moley") told me her moles were raised, dark, and even painful. These 3D nightmares were all over her body. She was afraid her husband wouldn't find her attractive and that her sex life would end. But in fact, the opposite occurred. Vicky's moles turned out to be a good method of foreplay. Her husband liked to play

connect-the-dots on her body. She said he once found a
bunny on her inner thigh that started off a rather nice evening.

All of these skin conditions, except for the moles, should
go away once you deliver. If the moles bother you, and your
husband isn't into connect-the-dots, see your dermatologist.

Backaches

"Oh, my achin' back" will spew forth from your mouth many
times during these next several months. I don't know one
mom-to-be who didn't suffer from this side effect of pregnancy at one time or another.

The main reason for the pain in your back is the bulge on
your front. All the extra weight in your tummy is throwing off
your center of gravity. To compensate for your hefty belly,
you naturally arch your back and push your shoulders together
hard, and keep it like this all day long (a.k.a., the pregnancy
waddle). The bad news is that this new posture of yours
pinches and strains your back muscles. The good news is that
standing this way stops you from falling flat on your face.

I wish I could say that this ache will get better during
your last trimester, but I can't without fear of being sued. I
can say that there are several things you can try to make your
poor achin' back feel just a little bit better:

1. Take a warm bath (remember, not *too* warm). This will
   relax those pinched muscles.
2. Put a heating pad on your back for about twenty minutes or so. Again, don't make it too hot. You don't
   want your womb turning into a hot tub.
3. Get a maternity support belt. It's a wide elastic support
   that's worn around your lower back and on the under-
   side of your belly. It gives your back much-needed

support and gives your tummy a gentle lift, which makes your back feel better, too. They cost about $50 and can be purchased through maternity catalogs or from ✐*www.maternityshoppe.com.*

4. Have your partner, or anyone else with hands, give you a good massage. There are actually professional pregnancy masseuses who specialize in rubbing moms-to-be. The best part about them is that some have a table with a hole in the middle (as well as one for the head) so you can lie on your tummy once again.

5. Sleep on a firm bed. If your bed isn't firm, put some plywood slats underneath the mattress.

6. Stay away from soft comfortable chairs. They slouch your back and can make matters worse. Besides, in your condition, you may not be able to get out of them.

7. Deliver your child. Although impractical at this point, it would stop the pain!

Sciatica

I thought things were going along fine. I'd made it through the morning sickness and the mood swings. I'd fought off fatigue and flatulence. But just when I thought that the worst was behind me, my behind felt the worst. I got sciatica.

It happened one morning as I got out of bed. I felt a sharp stabbing pain in my right butt cheek. To get rid of it, I hobbled around like an old fogy, hunched over and clutching my lower back. I half expected to see Willard Scott show my picture on the *Today Show*. The ache went away in a minute or so, but it returned each morning . . . *and* every time I sat still for any length of time. Being a pregnant woman, I spent most of my time sitting still for a length of time.

Sciatica is a very common pregnancy complaint. It's

caused by the growing kid pressing against your sciatic nerve, located from the lower portion of your spinal cord through your buttock and extending to your legs. It's one of the reasons that you can't sleep on your back—the weight of the baby can press down on it and do very bad things. (Sleeping on your back can also restrict blood flow to your heart, but since that doesn't make your tushy hurt, it's not much of a concern right now.) Sciatica tends to get worse as your pregnancy goes on because of the increased weight of the baby.

You can take Tylenol if the pain gets too bad. You can also lie down on the opposite side of the pain. If it hurts more on your right side, lie on your left. The only time to be concerned about sciatica is if the pain goes all the way down your leg. Then, you may be suffering from a disc problem in your back that should be looked at by an orthopedist.

One of the best things to do to relieve the pain from sciatica is to stretch. I took a prenatal yoga class where we spent a great deal of time doing stretches designed to help the tush nerve. In prenatal yoga, you use special mats and bolsters to contort your body into positions that you couldn't otherwise get into unless of course you're the pretzel woman from Cirque du Soleil.

In addition to helping with the pain of sciatica and strengthening the muscles used in labor, prenatal yoga class

> **❝** The worst episode I had was when I was walking across a parking lot on the hottest day of the year. I could only take tiny little steps and nearly got heat stroke getting back to my car. I felt like that old lady character Ruth Buzzi did on <u>Laugh-In</u>. **❞**
> —Greta

gives you something else you desperately need: a way to meet a gaggle of other pregnant women to compare and contrast your condition. If you decide to sign up, make sure the yoga class you're considering is a prenatal one, specifically designed for the needs and concerns of pregnant women.

If you're not into yoga, you can try what my friend Nancy's boss did when she was pregnant and had sciatica. She hired a personal masseuse to come to the house and give her weekly massages. If that's not an option in your area, there may be spas that offer pregnancy massages. I know that we all can't afford massages; that's why God invented husbands. Just give 'em a little massage oil and they'll rival any trained professional.

You can also do what the majority of women do—absolutely nothing. As good as yoga and massage are, the only thing you can really do to get rid of the pain is to get rid of the baby (deliver it, I mean). I was lucky. Unlike most cases of sciatica, mine had run its course by the beginning of the third trimester. I didn't tell my husband that, though; hey, I like a good butt rub as much as the next person.

Chapter Six

The Sixth Month

By now I had had it with the aches and pains. I came to the conclusion that pregnancy was just not for me. In fact, I was through with the whole reproduction crap. I started telling people exactly how I felt and that I was tired of being pregnant. I swore that the child that I was carrying would be the only one I would ever have. No *ifs*, *ands*, or *buts*!

But people just wouldn't get it. They'd give me that patronizing smile and say, "Every pregnancy is different. Maybe your next one won't be so bad." Yeah, right. How much better could another pregnancy really be? I'm still going to have to grow a child inside me and have it come out through the same exit hole. It's not like my next one would grow in a closet somewhere and I'd have to endure nine months of high cheekbones and dancer's legs.

People just love rooting for pregnancy. They'd been pushing for me to get pregnant ever since I said "I do." And now that I was, do you think they were happy? No way. And don't expect it to be any different for you. From the moment you push out your placenta, you'll be asked over and over again when you're going to have another one. It's truly amazing. The planet is full of pregnancy Hari Krishnas and the world is their airport.

Anyway, here you are about to start your sixth month—the last month of the second trimester. It's very sentimental really. It may even bring a tear to your eye (as if everything else doesn't). Enjoy this tear of sentiment, for in your next trimester, all the tears you'll shed will be caused by the sheer discomfort that lugging around a fully formed human being inside you can bring. But I digress. There are many goodies in store for you in this sixth month. I don't want to give any of them away and ruin the surprise. But then again, I guess that's my job.

Dark Back Hair and Other Icky Things

Believe it or not, pregnancy does make one aspect of your body better: your hair. Most women say that their hair grows in thicker during pregnancy. If you have thin hair to begin with, you're going to love it. If you have thick hair like mine, your hair will become a pelt. If you're redecorating, give yourself a trim and use the clippings to crochet yourself a fine area rug. But be warned, whether it was thick or thin to begin with, you'll lose this extra hair when all of your pregnancy hormones are gone. After you deliver, you'll brush your hair and large clumps of it will fall out. This could be rather scary if you're not expecting it.

Your hair might even change texture during pregnancy. My hair changed from curly to straight. Because hair grows pretty slowly (about half an inch a month), I never really noticed it until after my daughter was born. It was then that I saw a five-inch band of straight hair on top of my head. I had wished and wished for straight hair since I was in junior high when the Farrah Fawcett look was all the rage. After twenty years of hoping, straight hair was finally mine! But alas, when one miracle arrived (my daughter), the other miracle was taken away (my straight hair) and my curls returned.

If you're at all concerned about the texture of your hair changing, don't be. I have far greater things for you to be concerned with. For it seems that hair may appear in places where it never did before. It's as if your body is sprouting little Chia Pets all over itself.

You can blame the increased amount of male hormones in your system for these Chia Pets. Even when you're not pregnant, you have a small amount of male hormones circulating through your system. But now you have even more of them, and not only may you get more body hair, but you may also stop asking for directions and make empty promises to call the next day.

Like a man, you may develop a small patch of hair between your breasts, or even around the outside of your areolae. And don't be surprised if you sprout some facial hair. Perhaps a faint beard or a delicate mustache. Or maybe your eyebrows will thicken and grow together to form a unibrow. Now that's a *Glamour* don't! I have a friend who swore that the hair in her ears was growing. She also started to see more nose hair as well. Another woman I know from the park admitted that she grew dark hair on her back when she was pregnant. Luckily, with the new baby, she never goes out at night. I'd worry that she'd pillage the streets and howl at the moon.

You can bleach it or pluck it or wax this extra hair (if you're past your first trimester), but I wouldn't recommend shaving it because it might grow in darker and thicker (at least that's what my mom told me when I wanted to start shaving my legs). Just be patient. Giving birth will reduce your male hormone levels and bring out your feminine side once again.

Leg Cramps

It was Christmas morning. The whole family was gathered around the tree opening presents. I had just opened up a gift of ever-so-comfy flannel sheets. My husband wasn't as thrilled about them as I was because his body temperature runs about ten degrees above normal. It's like being married to Palm Springs.

Anyway, I was getting up to give the gift-giver a thank-you kiss and was instantly struck by a stabbing pain in my leg that brought tears to my eyes and me to the floor. Everyone in the room froze as they watched the landlord of their growing niece/daughter/granddaughter/great-granddaughter come crashing to the floor, screaming.

As a team, they joined together to move my blubberous form to a hard chair, not unlike marine workers carrying a beached whale back to the water.

As with almost all pregnancy pains, it came and left fairly quickly, lasting only a few very memorable minutes. The best way that I can describe the pain is either a dull rusty razor blade being embedded deep into my upper leg, or like a charley horse. And since I've never actually had the razor blade thing, I'll go with the charley horse. The rest of the day I was catered to and forbidden to get out of that chair. Even if you never have a leg cramp, I suggest you fake it. There are worse ways to spend the day.

Most experts agree that leg cramps are caused by either a calcium deficiency or an excess of potassium (but this is less common). If you're experiencing a lot of them, you can try quinine water that you can buy at most drug stores. Or you

> **"** I got a bad leg cramp once in the middle of the night
> and tried to walk it off, but my foot was locked with my
> toes pointed. I ended up banging by leg against the bed,
> which woke my husband in a panic yelling, 'Is it time?' **"**
>
> —Faith

can talk to your doctor. He may give you a vitamin supplement that may help. But the best remedy for occasional leg
cramps is heat and massage. I kept a heating pad by my bed
and a husband by my side. Between the two, all of my leg
cramps went away in a few minutes.

Leg cramps can happen anytime during your pregnancy
but tend to occur more often in the latter half. They also
happen more at night. Yes, I know that logic would dictate
that they would cramp up when you're actually using your
leg muscles, but they choose to strike when you've finally
drifted off to sleep.

If you're suffering from leg cramps and live in a two-story
home, I highly recommend investing in two heating pads.
Keep one in a central location on each floor, plugged in (but
not turned on) and ready to go. This will save you from the
ordeal of hobbling upstairs or down trying to get to one.

Belly Touching

Now that your stomach is starting to make its appearance in a
big way, the requests from strangers to touch it will soon
begin. I'm sure you understand how they feel. You may have
felt a belly or two in your nonpregnant days. A bulging belly
is a fascinating thing. Taut skin, stretched over a hidden
bundle of life. Touching it makes you feel as if you're a part
of the miracle.

So, when people asked me if they could touch my belly, I said sure. I loved to see their eyes light up. But eventually, I started to feel a little less generous. I would look at these slender women (they all seemed slender next to me) with their shirts tucked in, and, yes, I would get a bit jealous. Sure, I had a miracle in my tummy, but they were able to wear a belt.

So, whenever someone wanted to cop a feel, I had one condition. I told them that they could touch my stomach as long as I could touch theirs. Just as they got a thrill out of touching a belly with baby in it, I got a thrill out of touching one with an innie.

In conclusion, cherish the joy you'll give to others by letting them touch your stomach. It'll only last for a few more months. Or at least, let's hope so. My belly-touching requests continued many months after my baby was born, and believe me, when that happens, there's absolutely no joy involved.

An Itchy Stomach

As your pregnancy and belly progress, the skin on your stomach stretches and stretches like dough being tossed for an extra-large pizza. Because of this stretching, your belly gets really itchy. A pregnant woman I met told me that I shouldn't scratch my belly skin because it could cause stretch marks. Stupidly, I listened to her. She was on her third kid, so who was I to question? But as much as I tried, I just couldn't resist. It was too great of a temptation now that I had my long, razor-sharp pregnancy nails. Why is it that your nails get so enticing just when you're not supposed to use them? See, I told you Mother Nature has her cruel side.

I went to my local beauty supply store. They seem to have a product for everything, from scalp itch to toenail fungus and everything in between. I always find some kind of goodie in a beauty supply store and wonder how I ever lived without it.

I asked the lady behind the counter if she had anything for an itchy belly and she led me to an aisle that specialized in products for women in waiting. Imagine, a whole aisle! There was an entire shelf full of special shampoos, lotions, exfoliates, and other elixirs geared to the problems of the preggo. Most of these products were imported, which many people think makes them work better. Not me though. I went to Paris once and saw a box of Rice Krispies on the gourmet shelf. I guess they too think that if it's imported, it's better.

I'm a very cynical shopper anyway and decided to skip the tubes of the imported stuff, for some good old American petroleum jelly. Or I'd just slop on some baby oil or olive oil, or just about anything slick that came in my path. I found that most lubricants, from Wesson Oil to WD-40, worked just fine. Grease is grease, and whether it's cocoa butter or farm-fresh butter, it all does a good job.

So, when you're itchin' for some relief, buy cheap and buy in bulk. You're going to be using it for quite some time. And, if after you're slicked up like a greased pig you still need some more help, go ahead and give yourself a good scratch. I have it on good authority that scratching will *not* cause stretch marks.

Incompetent Cervix

Incompetent cervix, although very rare, is a dangerous condition that can occur in pregnancy. It's entirely curable but hard to diagnose. That is, until it's too late. An incompetent cervix opens up spontaneously during pregnancy and leads to a pregnancy loss. It usually happens during the second trimester. You could go in for your monthly visit and your cervix could be closed up tight as a drum. And then, for no good reason it opens up, causing you to lose your baby.

If you've suffered from a midterm miscarriage in the past, or any kind of cervical surgery, you're at risk. And if you are, your doctor will tie up your cervix and make sure that it stays that way until delivery.

The procedure is done in the hospital on an outpatient basis. You'll probably be given a spinal, so it won't hurt a bit (except of course for the pain involved in getting a spinal). If you know anything about sewing, you'll be interested to know that your doctor will tie up your cervix using a purse stitch. Maybe you can even request that he use a string in a coordinating color. How cool would that be to have your cervix match your handbag and shoes?

The one good thing about having an incompetent cervix is that it will excuse you from having to go to full term and endure those miserable last weeks of pregnancy (who am I kidding, the whole nine months can be pretty miserable). When you reach the thirty-eight-week mark, you'll be brought to the hospital to have your string cut and your labor induced. Things should go smoothly after that. Most cervixes dilate just fine despite the fact that they've been tied shut for months. Those cervixes. They take a lickin' and keep on tickin'!

What, Me Exercise?

You know you should do it. Your doctor tells you it's good for your baby. The books tell you it helps with delivery. Yes, they push exercise on you from the moment you conceive (heck, from the moment you're born). So, I thought I'd give it a try. I used to be in pretty good shape before I conceived. There was a time when I could run a 10K like it was only a K. I'm not gonna let a couple of extra pounds in my uterus stop me!

So, I stuffed myself into workout attire (which I found to be good enough exercise on its own) and headed off to my gym. I walked past those lithe-bodied athletes with my belly held high, and headed straight for the treadmill. "I could do this!" I thought as I turned on the machine. I started off just fine, with the stamina and confidence of the old days. But, after I ran what seemed to be the length of a driveway, I was exhausted. I was winded and nauseated and wanted my mommy. So I threw in the sweaty towel and went home, defeated.

The truth is that exercise is good for you when you're pregnant, but only in moderation. I read in one of my many research books that a pregnant body exerts itself standing still as much as a nonpregnant one does while mountain climbing. It's no wonder I got so tired. After reading that I decided to give my body a break, and if it seems best for you, you should too.

If you're determined to exercise, stick with the best exercise of all—walking. You should try to walk about twenty minutes a day and make sure that you keep your pulse below 140 beats per minute. If you're having difficulty talking and walking at the same time, you're pushing too hard and need to slow down. If you want to push your body a bit further, *and* you were used to pushing it a lot prior to becoming pregnant, go for it. But again, keep your pulse below 140! A consistently fast pulse rate may increase your body temperature, which isn't good for your baby.

The only other form of exercise I recommend for during pregnancy is called a Kegel. Kegel exercises tighten your vaginal and perineal (the area between your vagina and rectum) muscles and are good for a bevy of ailments from conception through delivery. They're easy to do and you don't need to buy any fancy workout clothes or join an expensive gym. You can do them anywhere, anytime. In fact, I'm doing them right now!

The way you do a Kegel is to relax your vaginal muscles as if you're peeing. Now, pretend that someone's coming in the bathroom and you have to stop peeing quickly. Can you can feel the muscles tighten? Hold them this way for about two or three seconds, then release. You should do about 100 of these a day (which works out to about ten at every stoplight). They sell expensive Kegel machines for hundreds of dollars, but don't be fooled. Mother Nature put a Kegel machine inside each and every one of you, and if you know how to pee, you're qualified to use it.

At first, I resented doing Kegels. They seemed like a lot of exercise without any visual reward. My motto is if it doesn't make me look better in clothes, why bother. But after reading about the power of the Kegel, I stuck with it. I read that it hinders incontinence and helps your privates return to a somewhat normal state after delivery. Some women told me that they prevent hemorrhoids as well as aid in delivery. Your husband will appreciate the benefits of Kegels too for it tightens up your vaginal walls after delivery making sex more enjoyable for him. I'm not sure if that will be a good thing or not, I'll let you decide.

Oops, There She Goes!

One of the things you'll notice around the middle of your pregnancy is that you turn into a one-woman slapstick comedy show. By now, just maneuvering your bulbous, waddling form around will become an act unto itself, and each act will include scenes with many pratfalls.

I was a constant source of entertainment. At home, I'd drop things all day long. I'd bump into coffee tables and chairs. In addition, I walked into a great deal of doorways. I thought I'd be moving just fine and then, bam! Smack into the door I'd go, headfirst of course. Now that's comedy!

The outside world would bring on even more challenges. I'd trip over sprinkler heads and cracks in the sidewalk. I'd often manage to fall into the street. Sometimes, I wouldn't see the curb, and other times I just couldn't coordinate my body down the six-inch drop.

I broke things everywhere I went. I was the bull in the china shop, the supermarket, the stationery store, and wherever else I went. Salespeople would give me a look of fear as I entered their shops. They were used to pregnant woman turning their display shelves into heaping piles of rubble.

There are several different reasons you've been transformed from a weeping willow to a weeping woman:

1. Your center of gravity is constantly changing. With your growing boobs, swollen ankles, and of course, expanding midline, you're like an acrobat trying to walk a constantly moving tightrope.

2. Your body is loosening up. One of your pregnancy hormones is called relaxin. It's a hormone that makes your joints, especially those in your pelvic area—you guessed it—relax. Because of this, your hips swing around like a hula dancer's.

3. Hormones are taking a toll on your eyesight. Not only is your vision not as sharp as before you conceived, but, if you wear contact lenses, you may be having trouble seeing because they've become too small. Yes, sadly enough, you're not only outgrowing your clothes but your contact lenses as well.

If you do fall down, don't freak out. Your baby is well protected inside you. Between the amniotic fluid and your strong uterine walls, the womb is one of the safest places to be. In fact, if you live in an area plagued with earthquakes, you may want to store your fine china in there as well for safekeeping. Even if you tumble down a flight of stairs, the only thing that you'll probably hurt will be your ego. Usually, only a severe force like an auto accident can cause damage to your little belly buddy.

If you're worried about car travel, you can buy a seat-belt adapter that fits onto a shoulder-strap seat belt. This adapter forces the lower lap belt to fit underneath your belly. In the unlikely event that you're in a collision, the lap belt won't push into your stomach, but below it. You can buy these seat-belt adapters through maternity gear catalogs and the Internet.

If you are concerned about whether a fall or an accident has hurt your child, look for signs. Has fetal movement decreased? Are you leaking amniotic fluid? If you're experiencing any of these symptoms, or you just want to put your mind at ease, see your doctor. He'll listen to the baby's heartbeat and maybe even give you an ultrasound. He'll make sure that the things that need to be attached in there are still attached, and he'll put your poor black-and-blue body at ease.

> **"I was a total butterfingers. When I got so big that I couldn't bend over anymore to pick things up, I'd walk around barefoot so I could pick things up with my toes."**
> —Pam

Here are a few things to do to stabilize yourself during these unstable times:

1. Don't wear high-heeled shoes. And by high-heeled, I mean anything higher than flats. Even half-inch heels are enough to throw off the whole body manipulation process.

2. Make sure that your shoes fit you properly. Some women think that their feet are going to spread when they're pregnant so they buy bigger shoes whether they need them or not. Your feet might spread—but then again, they might not. Either way, buy shoes that have a good snug fit. It's hard to walk around in over-sized shoes without slipping and sliding.

3. One good way to avoid turning yourself into a human wrecking ball is not to wear a large backpack. Stow it in your closet with your prepregnancy clothes and pull out a regular shoulder bag (large or small, depending on how much you need to carry). When you wear a large backpack, you become a danger coming and going. You're so conscious of avoiding belly contact with anything in front of you, that you forget about what's in back of you. Many times, I became a vaudeville act unto myself when I knocked something over with my backpack, turned to see what it was, then broke something else with my protruding belly. The only problem was that nobody laughed.

4. My last suggestion is that you may want to put away all the breakables around the house. You don't want to damage the family heirlooms before you even have an heir to give them to. Besides, once the baby's born, you'll have to put them away anyway. It's just one less thing for you to do as a new mom.

I promise that you'll return to your willow-like self after delivery. Your vision will revert back to the way it was before, and your joints will tighten up once again. Then, if something breaks, you have only yourself, or maybe your baby, to blame.

Pains in the Tucchus

Even years before I got pregnant, I was fully aware of the connection between pregnant women and hemorrhoids. I thought they went together like pickles and ice cream. But, luckily for me, that isn't always the case. Although I had plenty upon plenty of pregnancy ailments, I was spared this one (I think the third nipple thing filled my quota of maladies). The truth is that only about half of all pregnant women will get hemorrhoids. I've done my rectum research and, for those who really aren't sure what a hemorrhoid is, here goes.

A hemorrhoid is a varicose vein that's in your rectum (remember that a varicose vein is a vein that has a pool of blood in it). It looks like you ate a bunch of tiny grapes and it passed through you undigested. It's quite painful and can itch and bleed. Fortunately, there are some things you can do to prevent them.

The best thing is to avoid constipation, the biggest cause of hemorrhoids. All that strenuous pushing is tough on your tush. (See Toilet Troubles on page 75, for suggestions on how to avoid constipation.)

Also, don't lie on your back after about the fourth month. After that you don't want the extra weight on your butt veins. There are other reasons to avoid lying on your back as your pregnancy progresses, but avoiding hemorrhoids should be a good enough reason on its own.

If it turns out that you fall into the 50 percent of women who get hemorrhoids, there are things you can do to make them feel better.

1. Take a stool softener.
2. Put ice packs on the affected area.
3. Dab yourself with witch hazel.
4. Use topical pain sprays like the kind you get for bug bites and minor bruises.
5. Talk to your doctor. He may prescribe potions and lotions that you can purchase at your local drug store.
6. Take a tepid sitz bath. You can either take a bath in a couple of inches of water for about twenty minutes, or you can get the kind that fits into your toilet seat. The water seeps into your painful little nooks and crannies and takes the "owie" away. You should take several of them a day.
7. If you live in a walk-up apartment, move immediately!

I hate to burst your bubble, but even if you don't have hemorrhoids when you go into the delivery room, you may have them when you come out. You'll be doing a lot of pushing and straining and no amount of stool softener will be able to help you then. If you do get hemorrhoids while you deliver, the treatment is the same as it is above.

> **"My baby weighed almost 9 pounds and I had to push for over two hours to get her out. Because of that, I got a hemorrhoid. And even though it's healed now, my butt still itches every time I have to go pooh."**
> —Anonymous mommy

The other pain in the tail that may accompany pregnancy is a fissure. A fissure is caused by prolonged constipation. When you can't poop for a while, it builds up and becomes harder. So when you do finally go, your poop can actually tear a small slit in your rectum and this is caused a fissure. (Yes, I know this stuff is not your usual topic of conversation, but someone has to tell you about these things.)

Fissures can be quite painful. If you get one, the best thing you can do is take a sitz bath and use a topical spray like the one described. You should also avoid certain foods like corn and cabbage that are difficult to digest, for they may cause irritation. Fissures do heal in time. Depending on the severity, it could take a couple of days to several weeks.

The one and only benefit of having a fissure is that your knowledge of them may come in handy when your child becomes a toddler. It's not that uncommon for children who are potty training to get fissures. Kids can have a great fear of pooping and have an amazing ability to hold it in for what seems like an eternity. When they finally do go, it can take hours of screaming and pushing until finally, in one great push, your child will pass a poop that any trucker would be proud to call his own. And because of this, your little loved one may get a fissure. But because of your own experience, you'll know just what to do to make your baby feel better, because that's what a mommy is for.

Chapter Seven

The Seventh Month

ongratulations! You've made it to the third trimester! Even though you're into the homestretch, oh, what a long stretch it is. It's the "driving through Texas" equivalent of a trimester. It may only last three months, but that's twenty-one months to a dog or a pregnant woman.

For me, this last leg of the journey seemed to take forever. It used to be that all I wanted was a healthy baby. Now all I wanted was a baby that was *out of me*.

"What is wrong with me?" I asked myself on a daily basis. When was this going to start being fun? Was I crazy to feel this way, or the only sane woman in a world of pregnant Stepford wives?

I wouldn't discover the truth until my child was born and I finally ventured into the parks. It was then that I discovered that I *wasn't* the only woman who thought pregnancy sucked. It seemed that there was an underground world of us who suffered through the horrors of pregnancy in silence and shame. As Oprah would say, I had a light bulb moment. And this bulb had 1,000 watts and could illuminate an entire football stadium.

At the parks, we new moms would sit around the sandbox and bond over diaper rash creams and breast shields. And once the bond was established, we felt safe enough to finally purge ourselves of the ugly truth. Although there were *some* women in the group who loved every minute of being pregnant, most admitted to at least some difficulty. And there were others, plenty of others, who were as vehemently against the whole process as I was. At last, the words were spoken! Pregnancy can suck! And as they say, the truth did indeed set me free.

So, let me pave the way to enlightenment and be the first to say that it's okay to hate being pregnant. If you're having trouble reproducing, speak out loud and speak out proud! Let others know that it's okay to complain! Embrace your morning sickness! Share your gas!

And, while you're spreading the word to future generations of preggos, there are still more words of wisdom that I have to spread to you. For there are more attractions on the theme park of pregnancy. So hold on to the safety rails and keep your bloated hands and feet inside the ride at all times.

Swelling Ain't Swell

It doesn't happen all at once but rather creeps up on you slowly. First your breasts start to grow. Then your belly expands. But then, without explanation or warning, other body parts grow as well. Your hands expand like puff pastry. And your once delicately manicured feet look more like Shaquille O'Neal's after a big game. You're swelling up like the girl in the Wonka factory who ate the forbidden blueberry.

Although some parts of your body inflate due to swollen glands, a growing baby, or the extra weight caused by swollen glands and a growing baby, the rest of you is bloating because of your increased amount of body fluids. All that extra water, blood, and, in my case, Slurpees, takes up more room in your tissues. This condition is called edema and it's a fairly common pregnancy complaint. Edema strikes in various degrees. Some women may just get a little swollen, while others look as if they could float down Fifth Avenue in the Macy's Thanksgiving Day parade.

Edema tends to get worse toward the end of the day. It is also aggravated by warmer weather. Suffice to say, my heart goes out to you if you're a pregnant woman in Phoenix after sundown.

Sure, this swelling ain't too swell, but there are several ways to make you look less bloated.

- Drink more water. I know this doesn't make any sense, but I gotta believe that there was a study done somewhere that proved this method to be effective.
- Avoid standing for long periods of time.
- Wear support hose.
- Elevate your legs as much as possible.
- Don't oversalt your food. This may lead to water retention, which would be counterproductive.
- Wear comfortable, flat shoes.

I have two warnings for you. One, if you have severe swelling in your hands and/or your face, or if the edema doesn't go away in the morning, you should probably let your doctor know. This could be a sign of preeclampsia, a rather uncommon and potentially dangerous condition that should be treated by your doctor (see Toxemia: The Pressure Is On, on page 123).

My second warning is to check out your rings from time

> **❝** I woke up one morning and my fingers were so
> swollen that I couldn't get my wedding ring off. My
> dad made me come to his dental office where he
> proceeded to drill my ring off with a tooth drill. **❞**
> —Sylvia

to time. You should remove them every couple of weeks, just
to make sure that you still can. It's not uncommon for a ring
to need to be cut off a swollen finger so that it doesn't
impede circulation.

So, if your rings are starting to get tight, stash them away
with your form-fitting clothes, prepregnancy halter tops, and
other nostalgic items that bring tears to your eyes.

Temporary Insanity

It's downright scary that bringing a new life into the world
means killing off millions of other ones. I'm talking about the
fact that pregnancy causes every one of your brain cells to
die. At least if feels that way.

The process starts off slowly. At first you'll forget simple
things like returning a phone call, or knowing which side of
the plate the spoon goes on. But soon it gets worse. You
won't know how to work the microwave. You'll find yourself
at the office wearing different colored shoes. You'll forget
what the ingredients are for a B.L.T.

I'm all for women working as long as they can before
they deliver, especially if it means being able to spend more
time at home with the kid after it's born, but the lack of brain
cells can make this very difficult. When I worked, I felt sorry
for my employer. I can't tell you how many mistakes I made
over the months of my pregnancy, especially toward the end.

And I know that I cost the company some bucks because of my inefficiency. I only hope that my old boss doesn't read this book and ask me to reimburse him.

If I had my way, the government would pay women to stay at home during the last couple of months. Not to keep them from going to work, but to keep them off the highways. By the last few months you're down to just a few dozen brain cells, tops. By now, you've forgotten how to turn on the car. You mistake the accelerator for the brake. You think fifth gear is reverse.

I found one of the worst things about driving in my last trimester was how rude other drivers can be. I can't tell you how many times I was honked at simply because I stopped at a green light. I learned years ago, after I honked at an old lady making a left-hand turn from the right-hand lane, that honking should be used only in emergencies. I drove past the jerk and gave her the finger. It turned out that the driver was my grandmother. Luckily, she didn't see me, or anything else for that matter, above her dashboard.

Sex During the Third Trimester

Sex in the last trimester is like a jigsaw puzzle. You have to struggle to find ways to make the parts fit together. The standard positions don't work anymore so, unless you have the ability to defy gravity, you have to start using your imagination. Oh, and props don't hurt either.

I don't think I've ever laughed as hard as trying to have sex in the last trimester. There's something rather obscene about the whole thing, which also tickled my fancy. Soon, sex became a substitute for the Thursday night lineup. It was no longer a way to express our love to each other; it was just a way to get a good laugh without commercial interruptions.

As I mentioned before, my husband was never one of those who worried about hurting the baby when we made love. That was until now. By the third trimester, it was hard to ignore that there was a real baby inside me. I was able to see mysterious body parts pressing through my belly. It could have been an elbow, a foot, or maybe that big nose I saw on the ultrasound. My husband was getting a little more apprehensive. I think he was afraid he might create dimples where none existed before.

We did have one terrifying experience that I'll pass on to you in hopes of saving you from being as terrified as I was. It was during our anniversary trip when I was starting my eighth month. We had gone up to the mountains and rented a romantic cabin in a quaint little town. First, we explored the town, which took all of about ten minutes, and then we came back to the cabin to explore each other. (I'm trying to be subtle here because my dad might read this book. He's convinced that his granddaughter was immaculately conceived. Knowing what a slob I am he should know nothing about me is immaculate.)

As the exploration process was in full swing, I started to bleed. I hadn't spotted since the first trimester and, although faint, this spotting didn't seem to stop. All the panic of the miscarriage returned in a heartbeat, and I was terrified. Why was this happening in a town where the medical building doubled as the movie theater?

We tried to call my doctor, but it was a holiday weekend and he was away. We could only find a pay phone, which made returning our call difficult. I didn't bring along my pregnancy books that I was so dependent upon, so all we could do was wait. After about four hours the bleeding stopped. When we finally did get hold of the doctor, he told me that everything was fine. Sometimes, deep penetration during sex can cause bleeding. There was nothing wrong with the baby. I got off the phone and, with tears of joy in my eyes, told my husband the great news. Not only was he relieved, but he was also rather proud of himself. Men.

Toxemia: The Pressure Is On

I hesitate to even mention toxemia. It's not a very common condition as it affects between 5 and 10 percent of all pregnant women. But if you get it, it will certainly make your pregnancy experience suck so, therefore, it's worth including in this book.

Toxemia is the general term for pregnancy-induced hypertension. It encompasses both conditions of preeclampsia and the more advanced and serious condition, eclampsia. When a pregnant woman has hypertension (high blood pressure), it causes her blood vessels to constrict, decreasing the blood flow to her organs. Sometimes, this hypertension has symptoms. Her whole body might swell up like the Pillsbury Dough Boy. She may have headaches, blurred vision, and abdominal pain. Or, she may experience no symptoms at all (or ones that are hard to detect). For although excessive water retention may be a factor, there are times, like during the middle of August, when even nonpregnant women look like the Dough Boy.

The majority of toxemia cases are diagnosed during regular doctor's checkups. Your doctor will take your blood pressure (as he always does during an appointment) and if it's the magic number of 140 over 90, you'll win the prize of being diagnosed with preeclampsia. (Your pressure could be even lower if you had lower pressure to begin with.)

If your pressure isn't too high, you may be allowed to go home. If it's higher, you'll have to go to the hospital. In both cases, you'll be sentenced to bed rest and told to lie on your left side as much as possible. This can become quite grueling and makes simple tasks like twirling spaghetti quite a challenge (see Bed Rest on page 133).

With preeclampsia, it's crucial to try to keep your blood pressure within a safe range. If it climbs too high, you'll be at serious risk of turning your preeclampsia into eclampsia, which is a much more dangerous condition that could lead to convulsions or even a coma.

If your pressure does start to climb higher, the only cure is delivery. If your baby is close to term and its lungs are clear, get ready to be a mama. But even if your baby's not quite soup yet, it may still need to be delivered. A hospital incubator is a far less hostile environment than the womb of its eclamptic mother.

There is no way to prevent toxemia. Some say you can limit the amount of salt that you consume, but that theory has never been proved. Although the cause is still unknown, there are some things about toxemia that are known:

1. Toxemia happens more often to younger women, and ones like me, who are older, wiser, and able to pass construction sites without the fear of getting whistled at. So, if you're over twenty-five and under thirty-eight, you can breathe a cautious sigh of relief.

2. Toxemia is more common in first pregnances. But, if you had it with your first baby, you're more likely to get it again with subsequent pregnancies.

3. Toxemia almost always strikes during the last trimester.

4. Although toxemia is easily detected, if left untreated, it could damage your nervous system, blood vessels, and/or kidneys. It could also cause bad things to happen to your baby that I won't go into because I don't even like thinking about bad things that can happen to babies.

Third-Trimester Bleeding

Third-trimester bleeding is the technical term for bleeding that occurs during the third trimester. Although it is common to spot occasionally during the last months of pregnancy, it could be a symptom of several other conditions, most of which are caused by a placenta gone astray.

Normally, by the third trimester, the placenta has moved itself to the safe part of town, toward the upper portion of your uterus. But some placentas can be vagabonds. Even in your uterus, it's all about location, location, location, and where this restless traveler settles could result in some hazardous consequences. Let's explore some of these consequences that living in the outskirts could cause.

Marginal Sinus Tear

With a marginal sinus tear, the placenta has relocated to the very top of your uterus. I guess it prefers a womb with a view. What might happen, however, is that an edge of the placenta will start to peel away from the uterus. This peeling causes a minimal breaking away of some of the veins in the uterus, resulting in some spotting.

There is no known cause for a marginal sinus tear and there's nothing that can be done if you get one. But you will require extra monitoring and will probably be induced a bit early.

Placenta Previa

A more serious reason for third-trimester bleeding is placenta previa. It's caused by a placenta that's decided to hang low for a while. So low, in fact, that it may cover some or all of the opening of the cervix.

Sometimes, the placenta can just lie near the cervix without actually touching it. This is appropriately called a low-lying placenta. A low-lying placenta shouldn't cause much of a problem, and chances are, you should still be able to have a vaginal delivery.

Other times, however, the placenta may touch a small part of the cervical opening. This condition is caused a partial previa. With a partial previa, there's often some bleeding as the placenta starts pulling away from the cervix.

The third and most dangerous member of the previa family is central previa. The placenta actually lies on top of the cervix, between the baby and the vagina. With both the partial previa and the central previa, a vaginal delivery is impossible. Your kid couldn't possibly be able to pass though the tough placenta without some kind of power tool.

The beauty of previas is that they're easy to detect. Most are discovered during a regular ultrasound. But even if it's not, the third-trimester bleeding is usually a good tip-off. A previa bleed is as heavy as a period. When you call your doctor hysterically (as all pregnant women having periods should do), he'll probably give you a pop quiz. Did you recently have sex? Did you suffer some kind of trauma? Is there any pain involved? If you answered no to all three questions, you get the grade of "P" for placenta previa.

The treatment for previa with bleeding is rest. Not only bed rest but pelvic rest as well. But if you're diagnosed with placenta previa during your ultrasound and there is no bleeding, there's no need for bed rest or pelvic rest. (The only exception is with a central previa. If you're diagnosed with this, it's beddie-bye time for you and your pelvis.) If you have a previa but no bleeding, there is a small chance that, with time, the placenta will settle into its proper position and be no problem at all.

Abruptio Placentae

The most serious reason of all for third-trimester bleeding is called abruptio placentae. In this situation, the placenta has taken up residence in the proper place on your uterus, but then departs town like O.J. in the white Bronco. There are a number of factors that increase the risk of this sudden departure, such as high blood pressure, lupus, trauma, or drug use like cocaine.

There are two differences between abruptio placentae and previa placenta. One is the extra "e" at the end of the word "placenta." The other is that abruptio placentae is associated with pain. Although there will be some spotting, it will be the pain that will prompt you to call your doctor. At first you may think that you're in labor, but unlike labor contractions, the pain will be steady. Also, it may only be on one side.

Treatment for these two conditions is different. The good news is that with abruptio, you won't need to be put on bed rest. The bad news is that you will need immediate hospitalization. If it's discovered that just a small portion of the placenta has separated from the uterus (like 5 or 10 percent), the baby will be fine. But if the tear is larger (more like 35 percent), the baby will most likely die unless it's delivered.

Marginal sinus tears, placenta previa, and abruptio placentae are all fairly uncommon conditions and affect only about 5 percent of moms-to-be. And, although frightening, there is a bit of good news. If you have these, you'll almost always be induced before your due date and will therefore spend less time being pregnant! If that isn't a sparkling silver lining around a gloomy gray cloud, I don't know what is.

Braxton Hicks

Braxton Hicks contractions are the practice uterine contractions that you get during your last trimester. It seems that your uterus is like a professional athlete who needs to warm up before a big game. All of the books describe Braxton Hicks as being a bit uncomfortable, but I disagree. Unless of course by "uncomfortable," they mean like Hulk Hogan doing a body slam on top of your gut.

My cousin Amy told me that Braxton Hicks were no big deal, similar to bad menstrual cramps. I don't know what her periods are like, but I have never had a menstrual cramp that made my eyes roll back into their sockets. My cramps would last anywhere from five to twenty minutes, and I would get a couple of them back to back. Each Braxton Hicks episode could last up to an hour and would usually end with my losing my lunch.

Braxton Hicks usually begins about the seventh month of pregnancy and their rate of frequency increases each month. At first, my episodes were about three weeks apart, but by my ninth month, they would happen every week. Not all of my Braxton Hicks episodes caused me agony. But all were definitely bad enough for me to never, ever believe anything Cousin Amy says again.

The worst episode that I ever had was when my husband and I were on our anniversary getaway up in the mountains. (Yes, this was the same getaway when I started bleeding and when we finally named our daughter. We had quite the busy weekend.) We were just finishing up the breakfast part of the bed-and-breakfast experience, when I felt my stomach starting to contract. By the time I rushed back to the room, my uterus was like an accordion playing "Flight of the Bumblebee." I rocked and rolled for just over an hour with an encore throwing up in the bathroom. Braxton Hicks worried me so! If these were only practice contractions, I couldn't imagine how bad they'd be during the big game.

You may never get such intense Braxton Hicks; the vast majority of women don't. Yours may be quite mild like Cousin Amy's. But if they're not, here are some things you can do to try to stop the contraction:

1. **Change positions.** If you're standing up, sit down. If you're lying on one side, switch to the other. Do the hokeypokey and turn yourself around. That's what it's all about.
2. **Take a warm shower.** Warmth relaxes muscles, and when a Braxton Hicks contraction starts, it needs major relaxing.

Although Braxton Hicks are an inevitable part of pregnancy, you may be able to limit the amount that you get. One way to do this is to keep hydrated since dehydration has been found to bring on cramping and contractions. This is a good thing to do anyway. Another way is to keep your activity level down. I'm not saying to stay on bed rest, but it would be a good idea to pass on a day at Disneyland.

I Can't Sleep

I think that the hardest part of the third trimester is the lack of sleep. Before I conceived, I was a nine-hour-a-night girl. I never had insomnia. Never tossed and turned. Sleeping was one of my fortes. I even put it down on my resume under special skills, right next to my ability to say the alphabet backward really fast. But take that nine-hour girl and reduce her sleep time to about half, and watch her mentally wither away.

I was exhausted almost every day during my last trimester. My body was so weary after a day of schlepping itself around that it was in desperate need of forty winks. What with the incredible heartburn, Braxton Hicks, and a bladder the size of a kumquat, it made it difficult to fall off to slumberland. In addition, my baby seemed to have kick-boxing lessons through the night. And once the lesson was over, she'd hiccup for hours like a drunken sailor. Add up all these factors, and I was up half the night . . . if I was lucky.

I can offer a bit of advice to help you go off to la-la land. First off, surround yourself with pillows. They actually make a pregnancy pillow that's long enough to encircle your entire body. You can get these in stores, catalogues, or on the Internet. If you don't want to make the investment, use several different pillows around the house, and be sure to swipe your husband's pillow as well. Misery really does like company. Place these pillows anywhere you need support. I would suggest putting one pillow under your belly, one between your legs and a couple behind your back. Although this will give you relief from some of your aches and pains, it will give your husband very little room left on the mattress (which may actually be one more way to ease the resentment you feel from having to carry the baby all by yourself).

If you want a pill to cure your ills, ask your doctor about taking a mild antihistamine. There are several available over the counter. Yes, I know that an antihistamine is for a stuffy nose, but one of the side effects of an antihistamine is drowsiness and a good dose of drowsiness is just what the doctor ordered. Ask your doctor how often you can take them. Some will say every night, if needed; others will say not to take them at all. Some doctors are quite rigid about medication even in normal pregnancies, which is something I've already warned you about when it comes to choosing an O.B.

If you didn't heed my warning about the O.B. and find yourself awake during the wee hours of the night, here are things you might do to pass the time:

1. Catch up with a relative in a different time zone. Sure, you never had much to say to your Aunt Phoebe on the other coast. She may be dull and humorless, but at least she's awake.

2. Go on the Internet and chat with other pregnant women. I guarantee you'll find plenty of moms-to-be who are up, too.

3. Get extra cable channels. The best thing about being pregnant now versus when your mother was isn't the epidural, it's round-the-clock television with more than 500 different channels. When you're up all night, the shows don't have to be good, they just have to be on. So sit back and enjoy bass fishing or re-live great moments in golf.

Gestational Diabetes

Pregnancy can do serious damage to your body besides what it's doing to your waistline. It can cause you to become diabetic. This condition is called gestational diabetes and, unlike the type 1 or type 2 kinds of diabetes, its onset is caused by your offspring.

I didn't know much about gestational diabetes before I was pregnant. I knew that it had something to do with your body's ability to make enough insulin, and I knew that if you had it, your baby would probably be born big. And because a big baby usually means a big head, I knew that it was not the kind of thing that I'd be interested in. For that reason alone, I was a bit nervous the day that I went in for my glucose screen.

A glucose screen is the preliminary test to determine whether you have gestational diabetes. The test is given around the sixth month of pregnancy. It's pretty simple, really. You're asked to drink this cold ultrasweet syrup called glucola. It's pretty yucky tasting and definitely not the choice of *this* new generation. After exactly one hour (or as close as they can get), they'll draw some blood and measure your sugar level.

I never had a problem with blood sugar before, or sugar of any kind for that matter. Brown, white, powdered, or maple—I love the entire family. It's always been a good friend to me. It's comforted me when I was down, and entertained me when I was bored. It's given me support through breakups, and been there to help celebrate all my birthdays. And it's also my favorite movie companion. Luckily, sugar is fond of me too and I passed my glucose screen with flying colors. But my friend Emmy wasn't as lucky.

Emmy's sugar levels were too high on her glucose screen, so she had to take the dreaded Glucose Tolerance Test. It's three hours long and you'll need to fast the night before. You'll go in, have some blood taken, and drink twice as much of the nasty glucola as before. Then, you'll have blood work done one, two, and three hours afterward to measure your blood sugar levels.

Unfortunately, Emmy didn't do too well on this test either. Minutes after she finished her drink, she threw up in the nearby trash can. Then she blacked out. It's too bad that she didn't enjoy her glucola more, because little did she know, it would be the last taste of sugar she'd have for several months.

There are two levels of gestational diabetes, A1 and A2. If you have it, you should aim for A1. If you're diagnosed with A1 diabetes, you'll have to see a nutritionist and go on a strict low-sugar diet. You must also prick your finger several times a day to check your sugar levels, and pee on a stick every morning to check your ketones. If you're diagnosed with level A2, you must do all of the above plus the added bonus of giving yourself regular insulin injections.

Emmy was diagnosed with level A1 and was put on a diet that she referred to as "the chicken and grass diet." She could eat protein and most veggies, but no fruit, no bread, and only a limited amount of milk. This diet is incredibly difficult to stick with for a nonpregnant woman, but it's even harder for one who is. For not only does a pregnant woman have strong cravings, she also knows that no matter how closely she follows the diet, she'll never see the reward of a slimmer waistline.

If you're religious about your diet and testing, you should be able to keep your blood sugar levels in the proper range, and have a good chance of having a healthy baby. You'll get to have a lot more ultrasounds, which are always fun, and you usually get to deliver early. It's rare to go past thirty-eight weeks of gestation since the doctors don't want the baby to get too big. Surprisingly enough, a bigger baby doesn't always mean a healthier one. If a baby is like a bun in the oven, a baby of gestational diabetes is like a bun that's been left in the oven too long to dry out and burn. Ooops, I'm sorry. I shouldn't be saying the word "bun" to someone who has gestational diabetes.

Bed Rest

You can be trotting down the path of pregnancy and, for a vast number of reasons, be put out to pasture. I'm talking about bed rest. There are several conditions that would warrant a pregnant woman staying in bed all day. She could have significant bleeding in the first trimester. She could have hypertension, placenta previa, a decrease in her amniotic fluid, or maybe a risk for preterm labor.

My sister-in-law had low amniotic fluid and was confined to bed rest during her last trimester. I would call her from time to time to check in, and I'd listen to her complaints about how hard it was to stay in bed all day. I'd pretend to understand, but I really didn't. How hard could it be to lounge around in bed while being waited on hand and foot? I think everyone deserves a little less amniotic fluid from time to time. But the truth is, bed rest can be an uncomfortable, tedious, and often painful experience.

The amount of bed rest you could be subjected to depends on the severity of your condition. With some conditions—like mild preeclampsia, low-lying placenta, preterm labor, or a child who's small for its gestational age—you'll be placed on limited bed rest. With limited bed rest, you'd need to stay in bed (or on the couch) for most of the day, but you can still get up to prepare a meal.

But with more serious conditions like severe preeclampsia and placenta previa, your bed rest could be continuous. You could still get up for a quick trip to the bathroom, but the only meal you could prepare is Minute Rice. While in bed, you need to stay on your left side as much as possible. This position takes the uterus off the major vessels and allows an increased flow of blood to your uterus. Be prepared for misery, for although being in this position keeps the baby alive, it's going to make you nearly die of boredom.

Even though some women on bed rest admit that the first couple of days can be fun, it doesn't take long for the thrill to

"I used to hate sports and gave my husband grief for watching them all the time. But now that I'm on bed rest, I'm hooked on baseball. I haven't told my husband though. Whenever he walks in the room, I switch over real fast to the Food Network. **"**
—Vivian

wear thin. The truth, although hard to imagine, is that one can only watch so much television without getting bored. I don't quite understand the concept, but I'm willing to concede that there is that possibility.

After the boredom sets in, you'll crave stimulation. You'll mentally redecorate every room in the house. You'll create farm animals from the texture on the ceiling. You'll learn to speak Swahili from audiotapes, and knit everyone you know a colorful scarf.

The only place you'll be allowed to go is to your doctor's office for a checkup, and oh, you'll look forward to each appointment like a European vacation.

As you can imagine, it doesn't take long for bed rest to become both unexpectedly depressing and physically difficult. A body is not made to lie down all day, and after a while, it starts to hurt. Physically, your skin can get raw on certain pressure points. Mentally, you revert to being a kid. The moment that you're told you can't get out of bed is the exact moment that you want to do it. After a while, you'll revert even further. You become an infant who naps throughout the day and has difficulty sleeping through the night.

If you are put on bed rest, here are some things that you can try so that you'll be just a bit less miserable:

1. Get an egg crate mattress. It's a foam rubber bed that lies on top of your mattress. It has sponge rubber protrusions that massage you and take the pressure off key areas.

2. Even though you can probably take a shower, keep some premoistened towelettes by your bed. They're soothing and refreshing, especially those that contain alcohol.

3. Be kind to your friends. I know that you're feeling bitchy, but don't let it out on them. Your friends are going to be your saviors during this time and, if treated well, may bring you casseroles and tabloid magazines.

4. Avoid sad movies. Bed rest tends to make you even more emotional and sad movies can put you over the edge. It's sort of like listening to country western songs after a difficult breakup.

5. Buy a pair of walkie-talkies. That way you can stay in bed and still be able to yell at your husband while he's in any room in the house.

6. Do catalogue shopping for things that you need. Not only will this make you feel more productive, it will give you a reason to wake up each day. For seeing the UPS truck at your door turns every day into Christmas.

When you're on prolonged bed rest, it may take longer to recover after the baby is born. Your muscles may have atrophied. You have less aerobic capacity. But there is one possible advantage to it. Because of your weakened state, you may be able to get your husband to do more middle of the night feedings.

Chapter Eight

The Eighth Month

*A*s these long and arduous months have progressed, so
has the size of your belly. By my eighth month, my
belly was so large that I was getting nervous. I wondered just how big my kid was going to get. I considered
taking up smoking in hopes of stunting its growth.

But, as concerned as I was, I also felt strangely proud. My
belly stuck out of me like a moose head above a fireplace. And,
like the moose, it was definitely the focus of the room. People
stared at it constantly and I liked to show it off. I became a
flasher, lifting up my shirt to anyone who wanted a peek. I
showed it off to the neighbors. I paraded it around the dentist's
office. It got more "oohs" and "aahs" than the holiday turkey.

But the eighth month isn't all fun and games. In fact, it
can be rather frustrating. About now, you've given up
believing that your body is your own—because it isn't. You
may be the landlord, but your tenant has become pretty
demanding. He's made you curtail your alcohol consumption,
drug intake, and smoking. But you'll get revenge when you
do the same to him when he starts high school.

By the eighth month, the old "you" is but a distant memory. By now you can't stay up late enough to watch the six o'clock news. You can't cut your own toenails, let alone see them. You've given up shaving your legs and tying your shoelaces. You're having trouble getting out of a chair and can't last an hour without peeing.

In your last trimester, everything is hard to do. A simple walk from your car to the mall is now an exhausting journey. I think legislators should pass a law stating a woman in her last trimester be allowed to park in the handicap spots. If carrying around a human being in your guts isn't a handicap, I don't know what is. And, although you'd like nothing more than to put an end to your misery, Mother Nature, in her infinite wisdom and occasional cruelty, has a different plan in store for you.

Feeling Hot, Hot, Hot

So far, you've learned that being pregnant makes you vomit, swell, drool, bleed, ache, leak, and itch. Well, it also makes you sweat. Because of your pregnancy hormones and weight gain, your body's burning up. You'll find yourself perspiring throughout the day as if you're constantly giving an oral report.

It doesn't matter if you're walking in the snow, sitting in an air-conditioned theater, or swimming with the penguins at the Antarctic exhibit at the zoo. Your clothes will be covered with sweat (and possibly penguin dung if you do the exhibit thing).

Most women find this sweat fest quite uncomfortable. It feels like it's summer under your skin all year round. And if it really is summer, it will feel like you live on the sun. If your body temperature normally runs high, be prepared to sweat like a man with back hair. But if your body temperature runs more like mine, it may not be so unbearable. I'm one of those people who is cold all the time. I sleep under an electric blanket. I shiver during heat waves. For me, this overheating was actually a good thing. Being pregnant was the only time in my whole life when I actually felt comfortable.

Second-time moms are aware of this sauna-like side effect of pregnancy and some even plan their pregnancies around it. They use birth control in winter so as to avoid spending their last trimester during the hottest months of the year. If you didn't plan your procreation around the seasons, it may be too late for you. So, if you find yourself in a pregnancy meltdown, here are some things you can do:

1. Wear layers of clothing so you can peel them off as your body temperature starts to increase.
2. Sleep on top of towels so they can soak up your sweat. And leave some extra ones next to your bed to wipe off your body in the morning.
3. Take plenty of cool showers. This should lower your body temperature a bit.
4. Use baby powder. This will absorb your perspiration.
5. Get a neck cooler. They're kept in the refrigerator and worn around your neck like an icy-cold stole. You can get them at discount stores as well as fine gift shops. If you're too hot to shop, just keep some damp washcloths in the freezer and put them around your neck.
6. Come over to our house. My husband likes to keep the thermostat turned down real low so it's always quite nippy. It's a constant battle of ours, but we won't get into it while you're here.

Yeast Infections

Yet another gleeful part of pregnancy is the ever-so-popular yeast infection. Although there is always yeast in the vagina, being pregnant may increase its amount. It seems that when you multiply, so do they. Yeast likes sugar (as anyone who's proofed yeast for bread making should know), and when you're pregnant, you have a high sugar level in your blood and tissues, so there's more yeast.

I never had the good fortune of experiencing a yeast infection before I was pregnant. I'd see these women on television commercials talking about their new three-day treatment, and never thought a yeast infection was such a big deal. Boy, was I wrong.

When mine came on in my eighth month, I had no idea what was wrong with me. I went from feeling fine one hour to being so itchy the next that I wanted to go at myself with a fork. I had so much yeast in me that I should have doubled in bulk. I know women who have these infections all the time. How do they deal with them? And why weren't those women in the commercials going at themselves with cutlery?

Because I had never had a yeast infection before, I rushed to the doctor. He gave me some medicine and within an hour I was on the path to recovery. It was a miracle! Thank God for modern medicine and an O.B. who will dispense it. By the next day I was fine but kept a six-pack of medication with me at all times just in case.

If you notice increased itching or a thick cottage cheese–like discharge (now there's a pretty term!), it's no doubt a yeast infection. If you've had them before, you know just what I'm talking about. You don't need to go to a doctor, just to a drug store for one of those three-day (or even one-day) treatments. There are oral medications for yeast infections, but unless your doctor suggests it, you should just stick with the external medication.

Stretched to Extremes

One of the greatest fears associated with pregnancy isn't that of childbirth, it's the fear of getting stretch marks. Although plenty of women will get no stretch marks at all, many others will. Sometimes they're just faint silvery lines, but other times, they're so deep they look like the Grand Canyon. You could ride a donkey down some of those things.

Stretch marks are caused by a rapid increase in growth and, although they're quite common in pregnancy, anyone with skin is a candidate for getting them. Body builders get them because of their increased muscle size. People who have lost a great deal of weight can get them as well. So can anyone who has grown during his or her lifetime. My friend Allison—a tall, beautiful, naturally skinny woman—has them on her thighs. Interestingly enough, her stretch marks are horizontal, not vertical like the kind associated with weight gain. She got hers when she went through a growth spurt as a teenager. Secretly I'm glad. It's hard enough being friends with someone who looks like her.

I was convinced that I would get severe stretch marks because I was older when I conceived. I figured the older the skin, the less resilient it is and the less likely it would be to just snap back into position. But the truth is, it doesn't matter the age of the skin. It also doesn't matter whether your skin is black, white, red, or green. Stretch marks are an equal opportunity annoyer. What is important is the type of skin you have, and for that you should turn to your mother. Ask her if she got stretch marks when she was pregnant, and, if she did, tell her that now would be the perfect time to admit that you were adopted.

There's not a lot you can do to prevent stretch marks. If you don't believe me, you can do your own research. I'll bet that the only people who tell you otherwise are those who are trying to sell you something to prevent them. There is a vast array of products out there promising to keep your pregnant skin free of stretch marks. I've seen some exotic ones that contain sheep placenta and snail extract. I can't imagine that they actually work, but I do admit, I've never seen a stretch mark on a sheep or a snail.

Unfortunately, unlike most pregnancy ailments that we've talked about, stretch marks *don't* go away after the baby is born. They do, however, tend to fade over time. Luckily, stretch marks usually confine themselves to your stomach and your breasts so they're easy to hide from the public. Yes, your hubby will see them, but with the extra moles, spider veins, and broken capillaries, the stretch marks should blend in quite well.

There are two other areas of your body that can be stretched to extremes and may not snap back like they were before. These areas are never talked about except between the closest of girlfriends. One of these areas is your vulva. When they say being pregnant takes away your girlish figure, they know what they're taking about. I didn't do a global study; I just asked the few friends I felt comfortable enough to ask. But in all those cases, it was true. Their vulva skin got looser and dropped to a lower position. Maybe it happens when the baby's inside you or maybe when it drops into your pelvis during delivery. Either way, it seems that being pregnant may transform your genitals into gelatin.

The other mysterious area is your vagina. It seems that passing a seven-pound child through it loosens it up like an old cable-knit sweater. Some doctors will give you a "husband stitch" if you need to be sewn up after delivery. A "husband stitch" is an extra stitch in your vagina to tighten it up. Who knows? Maybe, like with your vulva, your vagina will never stretch out, or you may never be aware of it. And if your husband knows what's good for him, he'll never tell you otherwise.

Heartburn

You've probably endured your fair share of heartburn over these past several months, maybe even from early on in your pregnancy. In the beginning, heartburn was caused by the hormones that slow down your digestive system. Because your food stayed in your stomach longer than usual, it may have resulted in some bloating, gas, and, yes, occasional heartburn.

But now that you're in your third trimester, your heartburn is caused by your future offspring. By now your baby has grown to the size of a small chicken, and putting a small chicken in anyone's belly would no doubt cause some gastric distress.

The next time you're in your O.B.'s office, you can see what kind of damage I'm talking about. Take a good look at the pregnancy photos that are scattered on the wall. I'm sure there's one where the woman has been cut in half lengthwise, showing the internal organs, as if in a magic trick gone horribly awry. You'll notice that the baby is so large that it's flattened out her digestive system as if it's gone through a laundry press. It's a wonder that any amount of food larger than an antacid can pass through at all.

This is where my "long waist" theory comes into play again. If you have a long waist, there will be more than enough room in your belly to fit both your baby and your digestive tract. It's like having a piece of Samsonite luggage in there. But, if you're short-waisted like I am, it's like cramming everything into a makeup case.

My heartburn started in my seventh month. I was at work drinking my usual cup of decaf when I got my first inkling of what heartburn is all about. It felt as if I had just downed a cup of French-roasted battery acid. It suddenly dawned on me why they call it heartburn in the first place. It really does feel as if your heart is on fire.

During the next few weeks, most foods gave me heartburn. Soon, I had heartburn no matter what I ate, and then I got it whether I ate or not. I became a connoisseur of Tums and highly recommend the tropical fruit flavor. It's tangy with just a hint of tropical sweetness.

By my ninth month, I had acid reflux and could barely sleep. Whenever I'd lie down, the acid would creep up toward my throat. I would clutch at my chest in agony and feel the acid eat away at my esophagus, layer by layer. The only way that I could get any sleep at all was to sleep sitting up. If I was lucky, I'd get two or three consecutive hours— just enough to give me the strength to fight another day of pregnancy.

The old wives say that if a pregnant woman suffers from a lot of heartburn, her child will be born with a lot of hair. I, of course, was convinced that I would give birth to Rapunzel. I imagined her delivery to be quite entertaining. The doctor would pull her out by her long mane like a magician pulling out an endless chain of colored handkerchiefs.

There are some things you can do to avoid feeling the burn. Don't get too excited. There's nothing to take it away completely, but maybe the heartburn can be reduced to a heart singe.

1. Eat small frequent meals and eat them slowly.

2. If your doctor allows, try an H2 blocker like Zantac.

3. Get a pillow that raises your upper body to about a 45 degree angle. They're made for reading in bed, but they certainly help with heartburn, too. This would be the precursor to sleeping in a chair.

4. Experiment with your food to see what upsets your stomach. Most women are sensitive to acidic foods such as coffee and tomato sauce, but some can still eat spicy food without any problems. So do some taste testing and see what works for you.

5. Try drinking about an ounce each of aloe vera juice and black cherry juice together. This is especially soothing if the acid rises up into your esophagus. You can get both of these at most health stores.

Finally, don't listen to the old wives. As it turned out, even with all my incredible heartburn, my daughter was born with just a small tuft of hair. I think all pregnant women should pitch in and buy these wives some decent research material.

"Urine" for Even More Fun

If you look harder at that pregnancy picture in your O.B.'s office, you'll notice that her stomach isn't the only organ that's being flattened out. So is her bladder. And even though she's a two-dimensional illustration, you both have more in common than you think. For the weight of your dear belly buddy is pressing down on your bladder, too, causing you to race to the bathroom throughout the day. And not only during the day. Your need to excrete will wake you up during the night as well (if you're lucky enough to be sleeping).

Although these round-the-clock bathroom trips may be a pain in the tush, there is one good thing that may come from them. You'll get a lot of practice putting yourself back to sleep during the night. This will come in handy during the nighttime feedings that are just around the corner.

Although it's not a medical no-no, I recommend avoiding crowded public places during your last trimester. Not to avoid germs, but to avoid long bathroom lines. You know how it is—the men's room is empty while the line out the women's room is longer than the ticket line for a new *Star Wars* film.

Sometimes, the women in these lines would be nice and let me ahead of them. But others time they wouldn't. A woman with a bladder full of pee can be a very mean woman indeed. During those times, I would just use the men's room. Don't judge me. You'll probably use one too.

Luckily, there are usually bathrooms available everywhere you go, everywhere that is except your automobile. Although a car seat with lumbar support and leather upholstery is a good thing, a seat with copper plumbing would be even better. But I have a way to turn your Pontiac into a Port-a-Potty. Go to a baby store and buy yourself a toddler's potty seat. It's a portable plastic toilet that, if you're small enough or have good enough aim, you can use in your car. If that doesn't work, just pee in a jar.

Incontinence:
A Condition That's Sure to Piss You Off

By now, you're used to rushing to the bathroom to relieve yourself. But did you know that you'll probably be relieving yourself without going to the bathroom at all? Sometime during your last trimester, you may experience the joy of incontinence. In other words, you get to pee all over yourself. It's by far the most serious and surprising pee problem of them all, and one that I was never even aware of before I got pregnant. If you're not aware of it either, let me fill you in.

It seems that when you're pregnant, the hormones of pregnancy may cause some relaxation in your urinary tract making the tissue less toned. You may also have a more distended bladder because of all the excess pee. One or both of these factors can lead to pee spillage whenever you cough, laugh, sneeze, or even breathe.

It came as quite a surprise to me at first. I have quite a hardy laugh. In fact, I won "Best Laugh" in high school. It's one of my big claims to fame next to fact that I once went out with a member of *The Partridge Family*. Don't get too excited, it wasn't with Keith. It was with the drummer. Sure, he didn't wear a groovy puka shell necklace, but he still counts. Anyway, it seems that my best laugh caused me to wet myself during my eighth month.

I was at the nursery buying tulip bulbs. I had never grown tulips before because I thought it was too warm to grow them where I live. But, it seems that if you stick the bulbs in the refrigerator for a few months, they'll be tricked into believing that they've survived a harsh winter. This process intrigued me since I was feeling rather bitter toward Mother Nature and tricking her seemed like a good way to get even.

Anyway, I picked out my bulbs and asked the man behind the counter if tulips needed any special food. He told me they were rather fond of cheese pizza. He chuckled at himself proudly, and I gave him a zealous laugh in return, not because I found the joke so humorous, but more out of obligation. Then suddenly, I felt the leak! I stood there in shock, convinced that my water had just broken. I dropped the tulips, raced out of the store, and into my car. I got home and rushed to the bathroom half expecting to see the baby's head coming out. But it seemed that the only thing coming out of me was pee. I was disgusted. What was this pregnancy doing to me? I was being transformed into an old lady. I was forgetful, had bad eyesight, was in desperate need of a nap, and now had a crotch full of pee.

Soon, I peed on myself all the time. I peed when I laughed. I peed when I coughed. Sometimes, even standing up from a chair would cause the dam to break. During my O.B. appointment, I confessed to him that I had this problem. I'm sure it didn't come as a surprise with the wet spot on the back of my pants. He told me that the only way to deal with incontinence is to do Kegel exercises (see What, Me Exercise? on page 108, for more about Kegels). I, on the other hand, figured out other ways to deal with it:

1. Always carry around an extra pair of underpants in your purse and a pair of pants in the trunk of your car.
2. Wear panty shields. You may be doing this anyway for leukorrhea, but now they can perform double duty.
3. What about severe incontinence? Depends. Not on the condition, but *Depends*, the adult diapers. If the pads aren't enough, get them.

For some, this problem will go away after the baby is born. You'll regain control of your bladder and you'll go about your normal, potty-trained way of life. For others, the problem may stay with you. There is a medical procedure that can realign your urethra and bladder, but it's no easy matter. It will require surgery and a stay in the hospital. It will also take a couple of weeks until you're up and around and have your energy back.

Numb and Number

In addition to swelling up during pregnancy, your hands and feet may sustain another wound inflicted by the battle of gestation. But don't worry, you won't feel any pain. In fact, you won't feel anything at all, for this battle wound causes your hands and feet to become completely numb.

This numbness usually strikes during the last trimester of pregnancy, and it does so for several different reasons. One reason is that having hands and feet as swollen as Minnie Mouse's tends to inhibit blood flow. And without blood flow, there's no feeling. Numbness can also be caused by pressure on the nerve root in the neck. When this happens, the numbness may favor one side more than the other. Sometimes, this numbness is mild and more of an annoyance than anything, but other times it can be more severe.

One of the most severe types of numbness is called carpal tunnel syndrome. Carpal tunnel syndrome is the swelling of the nerves that go through a certain compartment of the wrist. This can produce weakness of the wrist and numbness of some of the fingers. And, of course, it can produce pain—a whole lot of pain. If this happens, your O.B. may refer you to an orthopedist who will probably give you a splint. Unlike heartburn or high blood pressure, carpal tunnel syndrome doesn't go away after the baby is born. It may last for a number of weeks postpartum.

I experienced a great deal of numbness during my last trimester. My hands had a habit of falling asleep during the night. I wasn't sleeping on top of them. They weren't twisted in any way. For no apparent reason, they just decided to go nite-nite. It was rather a nuisance. Although I was spared the intense pain of carpal tunnel syndrome, this general numbness did cause me a great deal of frustration. Not only did it wake me up, but I was also beginning to feel strong jealousy toward my own limbs. They were the only part of me that was getting any rest whatsoever.

As my pregnancy progressed, the numbness took over my whole arm. I would wake up without any feeling in my arm. And on top of that, I couldn't move the damn thing. It was as if I had a store mannequin appendage dangling from my shoulder. Was I paralyzed and just forget all about it? With my lack of brain cells, I thought it possible. Or maybe paralysis was just another side effect of pregnancy that I was never warned about. But a few seconds into my panic attack, I would feel a rush of blood pump back into my arm (I could actually feel it). The pins and needles would soon start, bringing with them my ability to feel and move my arm once again.

Oftentimes pregnancy numbness can strike during the day. And when it does, you may not lose sleep, but you might lose your grip. When your hands or arms are numb, it's difficult to hold onto things like spatulas and toothbrushes.

Legs and feet are prone to numbness, too. The main reason for this type of numbness is that there's pressure against your sciatic nerve. You may have a tendency to be a bit more numb in one leg than the other. You'll also have a tendency to stumble. But although you may act like Dick Van Dyke tripping over an ottoman, the blood flow will improve in a few minutes and you'll be back to your graceful Laura Petrie–like self once again.

Stop That Kicking!

Do you remember the good old days when you actually *tried* to feel the baby kick? I remember during my twentieth week doctor's appointment, I was scared because I had yet to feel the baby move. I, of course, was worried yet again that my baby was dead. My O.B. suggested two things. One was counseling. And the other was that I go home, eat a big meal, and lie down until I felt something.

I stopped off at my favorite Chinese restaurant and brought home some takeout. I wolfed it down, lay on the sofa, and waited. Then, finally, I felt something. It happened in an instant like a shooting star inside by belly. Was it a kick or just a gas bubble from all that slippery shrimp? Back then it was hard to tell the difference.

But as the weeks progressed and the kicks grew stronger, there was no trouble differentiating between the two. I'd feel a nudge and smile. It was proof, at least for that moment anyway, that my baby was alive and kickin'.

But now, even more time has passed, and your kicks are anything but delicate. In fact, they can be downright painful. What used to be a gentle nudge is now a swift kick in the ribs. Without warning, there's a jab to the right and a kidney punch to the left, so strong that it would give Mike Tyson a T.K.O. And this kind of internal fighting match doesn't just last the usual thirteen rounds. It goes on all day and all night. It wakes you from your precious sleep, which is definitely hitting below the belt.

You know why the kicks happen? Your baby is so cramped in its one-womb shack that every time it tosses and turns it causes you inward abuse. Although you understand, it still doesn't make it hurt any less. Isn't there some way to stop all this domestic violence? Not really. But there is one way to limit it: Stay away from concerts and action-packed adventure movies. Your baby can feel the vibrations and it kicks along to the beat.

Try to be patient. This kicking won't last forever. In fact, it will dissipate around your thirty-seventh week of pregnancy.

> **❝**I got married in my seventh month and
> I couldn't stand to be at my own reception.
> Whenever the band played fast dance music,
> I had to leave the room because of the kicks. **❞**
> —Ronnie

Before then, your baby has ample "womb" to kick around, and the strong muscle tone to do it with. But after thirty-seven weeks, there's less space. Sure, your baby might shift around in there, but it's too smushed up to really pack much of a wallop.

How the Hell Is This Thing Coming Out?

You can't put it off longer. The thought has crept into your mind several times before, but you were able to sweep it under the proverbial rug. But now, every time you look down at your gargantuan belly, you can't push the thought aside any longer. How the hell is this thing ever going to come out?

I've seen many wonders in this world that amaze me. One is watching a multiton plane soar through the sky. It's been explained to me that it floats on a cushion of air, but, like childbirth, it defies all sense of reason. I'm also mystified at a tiny ship built inside a glass bottle, but it's the opposite of the mystery of childbirth. I don't wonder how the thing gets out; I'm amazed how it ever got in there in the first place. But by far, the most eye-catching wonder is a woman in her ninth month of pregnancy. It's awe inspiring to see a human body stretched to such extremes.

The main problem with childbirth is that there is an inherent design flaw. There needs to be another exit hole somewhere. I propose that evolution create a hole similar to that of a toddler's pajama flap that snaps up in the rear. That way, when it's time for the baby to be born, the doctor simply unsnaps the flap, pops out the kid, and voilà! A baby is born. No pushing. No screaming. And cleanup's a breeze.

Of course, there's a great deal of fear associated with passing an infant through a hole designed to fit a penis. And, as much as past lovers would like to believe otherwise, they don't come close to the size of a newborn. So let's take a moment to ease some of your fears about childbirth. By now you may be asking yourself some of these questions:

1. What if my water breaks at a bad time? I can't think of one place where amniotic fluid gushing out between your legs couldn't be anything less than mortifying. But don't worry, only about 15 percent of women break their water before going to the hospital. And even if it does break, it should only be a few tablespoons' worth. And just so you know, amniotic fluid doesn't stain. So if you drip on your mother-in-law's new Persian rug, she should be able to blot it up with a clean towel and a simple spot remover. But, more important, even if you're embarrassed, you should also be jumping for joy. For the fact is that if you're full term and your water breaks, the clock starts ticking. Without that bag of water to protect your baby, infection could be a threat, so you can expect to deliver your baby within a day or two. Call your doctor and find out how you should proceed.

2. What if I can't handle the pain of labor? I'm not going to lie to you, labor hurts. I had a great fear of this myself since I don't have the highest tolerance for pain. I still shudder when I think back on how I rode out that headache without over-the-counter medication. But that's me. Believe it or not, some women don't find labor all that difficult. They must have the same genetic makeup as people who walk over hot coals. Maybe you'll be a coal walker too. And if you're not, there are always drugs.

3. What if I poop on the delivery room table? This is a common fear. Taking a dump in a room full of people goes against everything you've ever learned during potty training. But not every woman poops during childbirth. First of all, there isn't much eating going on during the final days of pregnancy. In fact, it's common to lose a few pounds. Also, while in labor, or maybe before it, you may have diarrhea or even throw up. This is Mother Nature's version of a high colonic, and should empty your system of everything but your baby. Also, by the time that you're ready to push, the baby has squeezed itself down to almost the end of the birth canal. If there's any poop at all, it should be just a dollop's worth that the nurse will wipe away without anyone being the wiser. If you want to avoid pooping while you push, visit the bathroom often in early labor. Even if you don't feel the urge, sit on the toilet and try to go.

I know you may have other fears. What if I need a C-section or an episiotomy? What if my baby is breech? What are my chances of dying? Childbirth can be a time of great fears and I found that the best way to reduce them is though

❝ I was pushing as hard as I could, but it didn't feel like the baby was getting any lower. Then my husband yelled 'It's out!' I asked him if he was sure, and he said 'Yeah! You just pushed out your poop!' ❞
—Debbie

education. Read books. Ask questions. Talk to family and friends. Soon, you'll become an expert. You'll know when you can expect your epidural. You'll learn how your doctor breaks your bag of water. You'll know exactly what hair accessories go best with a standard green hospital gown.

And most important, after watching and reading about so many deliveries, you'll be able to take a step back, breathe easier, and realize that after all is said and done, women have been having babies long before you. If it were really that bad, there'd be a lot more only children out there. So calm down. From a medical standpoint, there has never been a better and safer time to have a baby than now. I know for a fact that you'll have a far greater chance of being killed driving to the hospital than going through labor. Now don't you feel better?

Don't Breech to Me

By about the thirty-sixth week, your baby should be taking its proper position inside your womb: with its head down. Head up is called the breech position. If the baby doesn't invert itself before delivery, it can create a problem. A feet-first delivery causes stress to the baby and is a risk to your health. There is a chance that the head will be too big to fit through your pelvic bones and get stuck. Therefore, a breech baby, especially if it's your first child, is almost always delivered with a C-section.

But, fear not. Just because your baby is in the breech position now doesn't mean that it will be breech on delivery day. Oftentimes, the baby will turn around all by itself. And if it doesn't, your doctor may be able to do it for him through strong external pushes and prods. This external rotation can be quite uncomfortable since it requires a great deal of force. But don't worry. Although it feels like your doctor is treating your baby like Rodney King, he's actually not inflicting any harm to it whatsoever.

If your kid doesn't flip-flop, then you and your doctor will most likely discuss a C-section. If he does flip-flop, your doctor will give you a thick elastic waistband that will hold your baby in place like a large butt in a small girdle.

Chapter Nine

The Ninth Month

*T*his is it! The final month! The fat lady is just about to sing (or, in this case, scream in pain). If you've done your compulsive reading, you know that the ninth month is just a very cruel joke. By now your baby is fully developed and is able to live on its own outside the womb; it just needs to pack on a few extra pounds before doing so. I never understood why it just couldn't pack on the pounds *outside* the womb? We have Krispy Kremes out here.

You haven't slept in weeks. You can't stand another night of heartburn, and you're so big that you can't even fit under an exterminator tent. It's obvious that there isn't enough room for the both of you, and one of you has to go.

By now I've told you everything you need to know about common pregnancy ailments, so let's move away from that topic. It's not that you won't experience any of them in this final month. In fact, this is usually the most uncomfortable month of them all in terms of heartburn and sleeplessness. But, since I've already said all that needs to be said on those topics, I'm going to focus my attention on ways to pass the time during these last thirty days—as well as some info about labor itself.

Some of you might choose obscure projects like having a belly cast made of your stomach. The Internet is full of sites where you can buy everything you need to make a plaster mold of your tum-tum. It's a great souvenir from your pregnancy experience, and quite versatile. You can hang it on a wall, stand it on a pedestal, or lay it upside down on the floor as a bath for your newborn.

But for those of you who prefer to do more common activities, here are a few ways to keep busy during this ninth and final month.

Baby Shower 101

I hate baby showers with a passion. I'd rather receive an audit notice than a baby shower invitation. I started going in my early twenties and must have been to dozens of them. I played those stupid games, dressed in stupid girly dresses, and mingled with other stupid girls who played stupid games in their stupid girly dresses. I spent hours listening to women discuss when they were going to have a second child when I couldn't even get a second date. And then, after eating some horrible food, I would watch the endless barrage of presents that had to be opened one by one in front of everyone. And finally when it was all over, the shower-givers hand you a dorky thank-you gift as if to apologize for the torture they've asked you to endure.

So when my cousin Amy called asking me when *my* shower was, I told her that I wasn't interested in having one. Not wanting to put my friends through the ordeal, my husband and I were just going to buy all the stuff for the baby ourselves. How many things could an infant need anyway?

> **"**I thought we'd do something different and invite
> both men and women. But as it turned out the
> shower was the same time as some big game, so as
> usual, the men were in one room watching sports and
> the women were in another discussing diapers.**"**
> —Stacy

After Amy recited a list as long as a list of Kevin Bacon movies, I started to change my mind. I was amazed by how much it would take to keep a baby comfortable. She needed a special tub and unique handbag and an endless amount of clothes and bedding. It was as if I was giving birth to Zsa Zsa Gabor.

In the end, I decided to compromise. I decided that it was okay to put my friends through the torture of a shower as long as I gave them good food, alcoholic beverages, and by all means, *no games!* The main problem was that I had no one to throw the shower for me. My sister was broke, cousin Amy lived too far away, and my two dear friends were just dumped by their boyfriends and weren't in the most festive of moods.

In the end, it became a team event. My sister played hostess, Amy brought a slew of yummy desserts, my friends Nancy and Melissa did the invitations and cleaned up, and my mom sprung for some great food. I got the thank-you gifts, which I thought was appropriate since I was the one doing the thanking. I gave everyone a potted miniature rose, which was a big hit. I planted one in my own garden and every time I look at it, I remember the fun time I had.

To my overwhelming surprise, everybody I invited came. My friend Jaime even flew down from San Francisco. I obviously have friends who are much better people than I am. Each friend brought with them a wonderful present. I got everything I registered for and to my surprise, had a wonderful time. Maybe, just maybe, I'll venture to another baby shower one day. That is, of course, if they serve alcoholic beverages.

When it comes to gifts, you really need to register. Head down to your local baby store and they'll help list everything you'll need. At first, I felt tacky registering for so many things, but I figured I've bought enough baby gifts for my friends to raise the Waltons. These are the basics for keeping a baby warm and cozy:

- **Bassinet.** Bassinets come in a wide range of prices depending on the added features. I just saw one at a toy store that can actually vibrate (the bassinet, not the toy store). Personally, I hate bassinets but I know that many people think they're a must-have for a new baby. If you do get one, I suggest that you choose the one with the lowest sidewalls available (see Better Sleep for You and Your Baby on page 218). I've seen some that are designed to push right up alongside your bed that are good for nighttime nursing. They also make bassinet baskets with attached handles (often called Moses baskets), so not only don't you have sidewalls to deal with, but you can carry your bundle with you from room to room.
- **Bassinet sheets.** If you do get a bassinet (or are given one that's been passed down from generation to generation like I was), you should get at least two sheets for it so that when one is being washed (and believe you me, that will be often), you'll have at least one more to keep on the bassinet.

- **Diaper bag.** There is a wide range of diaper bags to choose from, from discount to designer. I've found that designer ones might indeed be stylish, but they don't always focus on the features that you'll need. I recommend you get a bag with a changing mat, a bottle holder, and a lot of compartments to store snacks, pacifiers, wipes, and the endless amount of things you'll need for that twenty-minute outing. I also suggest that you get one that's not too frou-frou looking. You're going to want your husband to carry it around at times and he may protest if it makes him feel too girly.
- **Diaper Genie.** It's a wastebasket for dirty diapers that keeps the stink in by turning the diapers into plastic-covered sausages. It sounds weird, but it's an ingenious invention. It may be difficult to figure out how to use it at first so I suggest you become familiar with it before the baby is born. Life will be stressful enough after that.
- **Diaper Genie inserts.** Plastic wrap to make the little sausages.
- **Receiving blankets for swaddling.** I recommend having at least five. You'll find lots of uses for these besides just swaddling.
- **Infant bathtub.** I suggest you get one that grows with your baby. I like the ones that have various ways to hold your baby depending on whether he's able to hold up his head or sit up.
- **Washcloths.** I suggest about six or so. Again, you'll want to have an ample supply while others are being washed.
- **Hooded towel for after bath.** You'll need about three. They don't have to be hooded, but if they are, your kid will look so darn cute!

- **Crib bibs.** A crib bib is another ingenious invention. It's a small piece of fabric that's made to lie across the crib. You put your baby's head on it and it absorbs the drool and spit up instead of it getting all over the sheets. You'll soon learn that changing crib sheets burns more calories than running a marathon, so anything that will decrease the amount of changes is a blessing. I suggest two of these.

- **High chair.** If there's not a big difference on price, I'd suggest getting a highchair with a reclining seat. This way, your tiny tot doesn't have to be able to sit up yet to use it.

- **Battery-operated swing.** Most babies love these. I'd love it too if it came in my size.

- **Bouncy chair.** I recommend the kind that has a toy bar in front and/or that can vibrate.

- **Stroller.** There are probably as many models of strollers as cars, so choose the one that works best for you. If you can't make up your mind, I do have some advice. Just as they say a woman can never be too young or too thin, I say a stroller can never be too lightweight and have a large enough underneath carrying basket.

- **Stroller toys.** They attach to the bar in front of the stroller and can make the difference between a screaming baby and a contented one.

- **Playpen.** Because my baby cried relentlessly whenever I put her down, I never used a playpen, but many people do. The best part about them is that they double as a portable crib whenever Grandma volunteers to babysit.

- **Infant car seat.** There are several different kinds of car seats. There's the kind that comes with a handle so

you can use it as a carrier. There are some that snap
into a stroller. Again, choose the one that works best
for you. Keep in mind that you should never buy a
used car seat unless you know for sure that it hasn't
been in an accident. A car seat is designed to with-
stand only one collision. After that, it must be replaced.

- **Older child car seat.** Once a baby meets the age and
  weight limit, you'll need to get a different car seat. You
  may as well register for this now. As before, beware of
  used car seats.

- **Gymini.** A Gymini is a colorful floor mat with toys that
  hang down from overhanging bars. You can lay your
  infant underneath it and he will be entertained for
  hours—or at least five minutes, which will still be
  wonderful.

- **Mobile.** I've heard that newborns see only in black
  and white (I'm still not sure how they know these
  things). I'm not sure if it's true, but I do know that they
  see better with sharp contrasts in color. Because of
  this, you may want to get a mobile with black and
  white hanging ornaments. This way, your baby may
  pay more attention to it and forget to cry for even a
  small stretch of time.

- **Diaper wipe warmer.** I know that this sounds like the
  epitome of luxury, but my baby would scream whenever I used a cold wipe. I guess she has a very sensitive rump.

- **Bottles and bottle accessories.** Nipples, bottle
  brush, bottle warmer, etc.

- **Childrearing books.** I couldn't get enough. As with
  pregnancy books, I found them to be invaluable. Please
  refer to the appendix for a list of recommendations.

- **Health book.** One of my favorite and most enduring

shower gifts is a child's' medical book. It is filled with all childhood ailments and tells a nervous mother what to do for every cough, sneeze, or rash.

- **Layette.** I found that the main rule for clothing a newborn is that it be easy to get in and out of. An outfit may be adorable, but if it doesn't have snaps down the legs, diaper changes are a nightmare. I also looked for soft fabric and snaps in the front. Because babies need to sleep on their backs, front snaps are much more comfortable. I suggest you get about five onesies (or T-shirts), three sleepers (blanket sleepers if it's cold), one long gown that ties at the bottom, two hats (one broad-brimmed if it's sunny, one tight over the ears if it's cold), bibs, booties, and mittens if it's cold.

- **Miscellaneous stuff, depending on your needs.** If you're planning on nursing, you may want to consider getting a breast pump. If you're going on a trip, register for baby travel goodies. The amount of baby stuff is endless and changes with every month and season. And don't forget to register for items that your baby will need down the road like bouncers to hang from door frames and toys for when they can pull themselves up. You'll be amazed at how fast babies' needs change and how many things to buy for them when they do.

Nesting Instinct

Nature has provided you with some wonderful instincts: the instinct to run from a fire, to seek shelter from a storm, to avoid fuzzy cheese in the fridge. But none of these instincts are as powerful as the nesting instinct.

The nesting instinct is where, usually during the ninth

month, a pregnant woman inexplicably and robustly cleans her house. I always doubted that there was such an instinct, so when it hit me, I was surprised. I know that I have some wonderful traits, but cleanliness isn't one of them. I've decided that there truly is a skill to cleaning a house. It takes a strong knowledge of household cleansers and an ability to work a sponge like a master craftsman. Whenever I clean my house, it always ends up dirtier than when I began.

But something happened deep into my ninth month that amazed me. I became a cleaning dynamo who adeptly worked a mop like a majorette working her baton. I cleaned everything in sight, and then cleaned everything that wasn't. I cleaned the back of the refrigerator, the high shelves in the closet, even the bottles in the medicine cabinet. I used dust rags and feather dusters and even old toothbrushes to get into the tiniest nooks and crannies. I was possessed. I was maniacal. I was my mother.

I wondered why it was instinctual to get the house as clean as possible. At first, I thought it was because my baby would be healthier in a pine-smelling, sanitized-for-your-protection environment. But then I thought of all those babies in rural areas crawling around through cow patties and they seem to thrive just fine.

It wasn't long after my baby was born that I realized the true meaning of all this cleanliness. It has nothing at all to do with killing germs or getting rid of that stubborn ring around the tub. The reason you clean your house from top to bottom is that once you push out your pup, you won't have time to do it again until your kid starts growing underarm hair.

It's been months now since my baby was born, and the layers of crud are rebuilding themselves like a city after a war. I'm afraid I'll have to conceive again, if only to get the house clean once more. I dread the day that my daughter will be crawling, and will undoubtedly ingest the hair and dead insects that have accumulated on the floor. I know that you're saying, "Just mop the floors once in awhile" and you're probably right. But then I think of those thriving babies in the cow patties, and I choose not to.

When it comes to the nesting instinct, the only advice I have is this:

1. Be prepared. Stock up on household cleaners. Get a new mop and plenty of sponges.
2. Hire yourself out to neighbors for extra cash. Believe me, this instinct is a powerful one and should be used for good.
3. Because of the dangerously strong fumes, stay away from toxic solvents like oven cleaners and bug spray.

Lamaze Class

Lamaze class has two important functions. One is to educate you in all aspects of labor and delivery. The other is to pass the time during this endless and uncomfortable last month. Don't underestimate the importance of the second function.

There are lots of Lamaze classes available and several different ways to find them. You could ask your doctor for a recommendation. You could ask the hospital where you're going to deliver, or you could ask a friend or family member who went to one. But be warned, even though there are many classes to take, you usually need to sign up several weeks in advance in order to take it. The classes last about six weeks and you shouldn't start a class when you're more than thirty-two weeks along. It'd be frustrating to go into labor without learning how to breathe through a contraction.

If you don't have the time or the desire to attend classes

for six weeks, there are private Lamaze lessons available. They're more expensive but take far less time. They can be completed in less than one weekend. My husband and I decided to go with the public class and I'm glad that we did. It met every Tuesday night and I started to look forward to Tuesdays like a prisoner awaiting a conjugal visit. I'd mark my calendar and get all dressed up (which means that I wore an outfit without any stains on the boob area).

Our class was given by a labor and delivery nurse and the meetings took place at her home. There were seven other couples in our group and we bonded instantly. Not since detention did I find a class with people all going through the same experience at the same time.

I learned many things in Lamaze class. I learned that there are actually three stages of labor: latent, active, and advanced. I learned how to breathe so I could manage the pain of contractions. But by far the most important thing I learned in my Lamaze class is that there truly is someone for everyone. I met some of the weirdest couples I'd ever met in that class, and the fact that they were reproducing scared me to death. There was one man in particular who disturbed me the most. Whenever he'd raise his hand to ask a question, I would cringe. For instance, he asked what kind of cereal he should feed his child once it started on solid foods. Granola, bran flakes, or what? Sometimes, I'll think about the infant born to this strange man, and hope that it's doing okay. Is it dressed warmly? Is it being sung to sleep? Did it choke on a spoonful of Fruity Pebbles?

Lamaze class teaches you other pointers as well. There was one class where we learned how to push. You'd think that pushing would be easy, especially after all those months of constipation, but there is actually a right way and a wrong way to push (we'll get to that later). Lamaze classes will also teach you when it's time to go to the hospital, and you'll probably be given a lesson on breastfeeding (more on that stuff later, too). But best of all, you get to see a film! Be prepared because some of it can get pretty graphic. It's like watching the film *Red Asphalt* from driving school. The film we saw showed an actual delivery and it was pretty nasty. It could have doubled as an ad for birth control.

Although many people will tell you that Lamaze class is a waste of time, I still recommend that you go. Some say that they never used anything they learned at Lamaze especially if you plan to have an epidural to knock out your sense of pain. I still think that the classes are worth taking. I don't want to scare you (although I guess this entire book probably makes you a bit nervous), but just because you want an epidural doesn't always mean that you're going to get one. And besides, even if you do get an epidural, you'll have some early contractions to deal with—plus you still need something to do on Tuesday nights. If you do decide to take the class, here are some tips:

1. Bring nice pillows. You're going to be asked to bring your pillows with you, and your pillowcases will be more of a status symbol than the car you used to drive to class. I'm not saying to go out and invest in a set of Shabby Chics, but don't bring your "I Sleep with Stupid" with a pointed arrow set either.

2. Bring paper and pen. This isn't to jot down important labor information, but rather to get a classmate's phone number. Lamaze class is like Club Med for the expecting. I know several people who still "date" other couples they met in Lamaze.

3. If you're finding that the classes are making you more nervous about your pending delivery, stop taking them. There are times when ignorance is bliss.

There are other natural birthing classes available, such as the Bradley Method. Like Lamaze, the Bradley Method focuses on breathing techniques to manage the pain, but it also emphasizes diet and exercise. In general, most all birthing classes stress the use of pain management versus pain killers during labor. Learn about the different classes that are available in your area and choose the one that's right for you.

Nursing Bras

I was told that I should wait until the ninth month to buy my nursing bras because, by then, my breasts would be as big as they were ever going to get. WRONG. As enormous as they were in the ninth month, it was a preview of coming attractions. But even though your boobs may still grow bigger, I still suggest that you buy your nursing bras now.

The main reason for buying them before your milk comes in is that you aren't going to feel much like doing it afterward. Somehow fresh stitches in your genitalia combined with engorged leaky breasts and severe sleep deprivation can take all the fun out of walking around a mall for hours on end. New moms take the term "shop till you drop" quite literally.

When you do shop, I suggest that you go to a place that specializes in nursing bras. A trained saleswoman will be able to look at you and estimate the size you'll need once your milk comes in. I didn't go to a specialty store. The saleswoman

❝I bought a couple of nursing bras and didn't even know it. I don't even have any kids. I just saw them at the store and thought the flap was kind of sexy. ❞
—Debra

who helped didn't have much experience with lactating bosoms and advised me to buy a bra with an underwire. She said that underwires offer good support, and since I had the weight of toaster ovens dangling from my chest, this sounded like an important feature. It wasn't until later on that I found out that underwires give your breasts clogs as well as support. A nursing expert told me that the wires tend to push in on your milk ducts and obstruct their flow.

Another important quality in a nursing bra is that you should be able to fasten it together with only one hand. Personally, I prefer the kind of bra that simply crosses over in the front without any snaps whatsoever. They also sell the kind that snaps up in front at the center. I found these types to be the easiest to operate as well as the most discreet. The bras that hook together at the top of the front strap were difficult for me to master. It took me almost three months, approximately 520 feedings, before I could get my boobs back inside them using only one hand. I now know what an Olympic athlete goes through to make their chosen sport look so easy.

When buying your bras, bear this in mind:

1. Buy at least three of them. You'll need one to wear, one for your drawer, and one for the laundry.
2. Don't be cheap. These bras have a lot of lifting and supporting to do, so I suggest that you get ones that are well made.
3. If you already bought some that are underwire, take out the wire. Cut a little slit at the top part of the bra and they should just slide right out. You can use the underwire for a good game of horseshoes.

Decorating the Baby's Room

Don't worry. I'm not going to give you decorating advice. I don't know a duvet from a bidet. But I do know that now would be a good time to get the baby's room in order. I know this sounds obvious, but many people don't decorate the room until the baby is born. Some people think it's bad luck. Others think they'll have free time once the baby comes home. Some want to see the sex of the child first. But I recommend doing as much as you can now.

Keep in mind that when you get back from the hospital, you probably won't be able to drive right away. I wasn't allowed to get behind a wheel for two weeks. And even when I could drive again, my pediatrician said I couldn't take the baby into crowded places for four to six weeks. It's hard to get baby stuff at a place that's not crowded.

Even once you can drive, it's hard to drive with a newborn. The poor kid can't hold its neck up. It flops around in the infant seat like a sock puppet. They only make rear-facing infant seats so you can't see the poor tyke boppin' and a rollin'. My baby cried all the time when I drove, and I couldn't tell if she was just being fussy or if I broke her neck on the last U-turn.

Decorating a room can take quite a lot of time and research. I went to the three local baby stores in my area and browsed their shops and catalogues. It was also a long discussion with the hubby as to what the color scheme should be. I wanted pastels; he wanted browns (I still think he wasn't convinced it was a girl). Needless to say, we went with the pastels. After all, he got to pick the name that she's going to have for her entire life. The least that I could do was pick out her sheets.

Since it was going to be our first—and I was convinced our *only*—child, we went all out. We bought a handmade rug. My sister and I made curtains with a sweet floral print. We got an antique rocking chair that one day our baby can use to nurse her own child. I really liked the way the room came out and enjoyed the fact that I could decorate it the way that I wanted. I know one day she'll replace the print of Beatrix Potter with one of Harry Potter, but for now, I'm running the show.

Obviously, decorating a baby's room is a very personal matter. I wouldn't begin to tell you what colors to choose, but I would begin to give you some suggestions:

1. If you're going to paint the room, don't do it yourself. Pregnant women aren't supposed to breathe paint fumes for any length of time. My husband was in charge of painting and did all the work himself. This eased some of the resentment I had toward him for not having to sleep in a chair.

2. Believe it or not, the least important item in a baby's room is the crib. For the first three months or so, you're probably going to want the baby to sleep with you in your room. It will be easier to feed it and keep an eye on it if it's nearby. You may want to keep it in a bassinet, in your bed, or maybe even your sock drawer (you laugh if this is your first kid, but you'll say "good idea" if it's your second). So, if you can't decide which crib to choose, or if it won't come in until after your baby comes out, don't freak.

3. Get a changing table with plenty of storage room. Changing a baby's diaper entails a great deal of paraphernalia and no matter how cute the changing table may be, pass on it if it doesn't have storage. They sell changing tables separately or have the kind that're built on top of a chest of drawers.

Taking a Tour of the Hospital

Most hospitals offer a tour of the maternity ward on a weekly or monthly basis, and I highly suggest that you go on one. Not only will this give you a chance to acquaint yourself with the place, it also allows you to perform a crucial bit of business: preregistration.

Although you should check with your hospital, you can probably preregister anytime within a couple of months of your due date. But if you were the kind of kid who put off weekend homework assignments until Monday morning, this last-minute opportunity is for you. No matter when you do it, you *should* preregister. It won't be much fun to search for your insurance card with amniotic fluid dripping down your legs.

The first thing you'll want to check out is where to park on delivery day. Most hospitals have specific places during an emergency such as this and you should know it in advance. You'd hate to have your husband abandon you in the heat of labor in order to repark the car.

Of course, you'll also want to see the labor rooms and familiarize yourself with the equipment inside, the most important of which will be the phone. Find out how to make a call. Do you just have to dial out or do you need a calling card? And if there's not a phone in your room, where is the closest pay phone you can use? And remember to bring a roll of quarters with you on delivery day. If you have a cell phone, delivery day would be a good day to carry it with you.

You should also find out about the epidural procedure. Getting an epidural isn't always as easy as just asking for it. Your hospital may have just one anesthesiologist who gives them and many deserving women. There may be tests that need to be performed beforehand that may take some time. You want to know all of this now, not when you're writhing in pain.

You should also check out the labor bed. You may have a certain delivery position in mind and you'll want to make sure that the bed is equipped with whatever equipment you may need. You may want handrails or a bed that can contort into a certain position. Now is the time to check for those things.

While you're in the room, you may notice that there is no closet. I point this out because people have a habit of packing for labor like they're packing for a vacation. They bring clothing, pillows, pictures, CD players, and even a cooler. As you can imagine, there's no place to put all this stuff. You're in an interim labor room, not a cabin at the lake.

While you're at the hospital, you should peep in on the nursery. We did and saw several precious newborns who were delivered just moments before. Seeing those shriveled-up little miracles reminded me that pregnancy was about more than just getting seated quickly at a crowded restaurant.

On the day of your tour, listen to what the guide has to say and check out everything you can. You're going to be a paying guest and should know about their accommodations. Is there a shower? Do they have a lactation specialist available to help you with the first breastfeeding? Don't be intimidated or embarrassed to ask questions. If, for whatever reasons, you don't like the hospital where your doctor delivers, talk to him about it. He may have hospital privileges elsewhere—though he may be reluctant to use them because of the logistical difficulties of having women in labor at different locations.

Taking a tour of the hospital can be quite educational, and a great deal of fun. It's exciting to see the room where you'll deliver your baby, and to know that soon, you'll be screaming in pain with the rest of them. But it was exciting for me for a different reason, for I won the hospital raffle! It was the first time in my life that I ever won anything. Sure, it was only a sample of iron-rich formula, but it couldn't have been more exciting if Ed McMahon rang my doorbell on SuperBowl Sunday.

Am I in Labor?

During the ninth month, you're on "delivery high alert." You're sensitive to every minute sensation your body has to offer. Was that a labor pain or Braxton Hicks? Is that bloody show or just some spotting? Did my water break or did I just pee all over myself again? There are some signs that could mean the beginning of labor. You may get them or you may not. But you should at least know what to look for.

- Your mucous plug becomes dislodged. The mucous plug is just that: a plug made out of mucous. It's spent the last nine months corking up your cervix to protect your baby from infection. This could happen the day of delivery or up to two weeks beforehand. You might pass this plug all in one piece, or, as in most cases, it may disintegrate slowly.
- You may experience an increase in your lower back pain.
- You may become nauseated.
- You may experience some pressure on the interior part of your thighs.
- You may lose your appetite.
- Your vaginal fluid may become thicker.
- You may begin to have a bloody show. This occurs when your cervix starts to dilate causing the capillaries

in it to break. This leads to bloody secretions that signify the onset of labor.

- You may have stomach distress that may clean out your system. Soon all your body's energy must go into excreting a baby, not digesting a tuna melt.
- Your water breaks. This is the most definite sign that labor is about to begin.

If you're experiencing these symptoms, you may be in early labor. Stay at home until you're sure (if your water breaks, ask your doctor whether he feels you should stay at home or go to the hospital). Wait until you have twelve baby-making contractions in an hour before you arrive at the hospital (a baby-making contraction is one that's so bad that you have trouble talking through it).

I know that the standard rule of thumb is to go to the hospital when the contractions are five minutes apart, but that's not true in every case. I live in a crowded city with heavy rush hour traffic. A ten-minute car ride to the hospital with no traffic could easily take three times that long during heavy congestion. If you have that situation, or just live far from the hospital, try to leave in time so that you can *get* to the hospital when the contractions are five minutes apart.

And keep in mind, if this is your second or third baby, you'll need to get to the hospital even earlier. In general, the first kid takes the longest to come out. They must leave a trail of bread crumbs behind in your vagina because the next kids find their way out in a fast and feverish manner.

My opinion is that you should stay at home as long as possible. You may not want to get to the hospital before you need to. Once you've been checked in, you're in their control, and hospitals have strict guidelines to follow. You may want to wander around the halls, but, if it's warranted, they may need you in bed attached to a fetal monitor or an IV. Once you enter their ballpark, you have to play by their rules.

False Labor

As if it weren't frustrating enough to figure out when labor begins, there's something else to be aware of toward the end of pregnancy: false labor. I fell prey to this evil savage myself.

One night in my thirty-eighth week, I woke up with what I thought were Braxton Hicks contractions. But after a little time I realized that the cramping felt different from my usual Braxton Hicks episodes. I would get a cramp that would last just a few minutes and then go away. And, I felt no pain in between the contractions. After about twenty minutes, another contraction would set in and it would last for about the same amount of time. This went on for a couple of hours and I thought I was finally in labor! Zippity doo dah!

I woke up my husband and we started timing the contractions. But after about two hours, the cramps stopped completely. I wasn't in labor. Now I was thinking something much more crude, more from a Martin Lawrence movie than a Disney film.

The next morning I called my doctor and told him what happened. He said that in fact, I was in labor but that it had stalled (a.k.a. false labor). He described my uterus as being like a car engine on a cold morning. Sometimes, it just doesn't get going the first time.

One of the main reasons for false labor is that you're so damn sick of being pregnant that even the slightest twinge could mean the beginning of the end. You may read more into each ping and pang because you want to be in labor so badly, but wishing just won't make it come true. There are definite distinctions between real labor pains and false ones. Real labor pains:

- Occur at decreasing intervals
- Are strong and increase in strength
- Don't subside if you move around
- Don't go away after a couple of hours

Although deflating, false labor should give you hope. It means that soon your uterus won't stall. It will rev up like a Porsche and drive itself right to the emergency ward.

How to Start Labor

I bet by now you're going out of your mind. Not only do you want to put an end to your pregnancy, you want to put an end to the constant barrage of phone calls asking if you're in labor yet. I know I was tired of it all. I tried everything I could to start labor. I jumped up and down, and pushed down hard on my stomach. I did everything shy of sticking my hand up myself and yanking the kid out. Wasn't there any way to get this thing out of me?

Although I wasn't sure of a good way to start labor, I did know of a bad way. *Do not try to start labor with nipple stimulation!* You may have heard that this trick works, but it's a very dangerous thing to do. Even though it might cause contractions, the kind that it could cause are called tetanic contractions. They could last ten minutes instead of the usual forty-five seconds, and they can be extremely dangerous to the baby. I'm not saying you (or invited guests) can't touch your breasts, just don't put your fingers on your nipples and rub them together for any length of time.

So, just like with morning sickness, I thought I'd turn to the experts (new moms) for suggestions on how to start labor safely. Just as with morning sickness, none of the suggestions worked for me, but I'll pass them on to you anyway in hopes that they'll do the trick:

1. Take a walk. By far, the number one method that was advised to me was to take a long walk. I met a woman who walked a couple of miles every morning and, not only did she say that she delivered early, but she credited this method for "a delivery as painless as a bikini wax."

2. Take castor oil. This is an old-fashioned remedy that many people swear by. I don't believe in it myself. I bet that the only thing you'll deliver after taking castor oil is a seven-pound bowel movement.

3. Eat spicy food. I hate spicy food but nonetheless ate it quite often during the end of my pregnancy. Afterward, I would lie still and wait for the painful contractions to begin. Unfortunately, the only pains I experienced were the pain of my stomach lining being eaten away by all the heartburn caused by the spicy food. If you're susceptible to heartburn, I recommend you skip this method. A stomach lining is a terrible thing to waste.

4. Exercise mind over matter. I was told that your mind has a great deal of control over what happens to your body. If you concentrate hard enough, you can alter the rate of your heartbeat and your breathing. So I figured if I concentrated hard enough, I could get my body to start labor. I envisioned the contractions. I imagined my cervix opening up. I mentally ordered every cell in my womb to start to push. But in the end I gave up. I decided it would have been easier to bend a spoon with my mind then get it to start labor.

5. Have sex. Unlike the other methods, medical science backs this one. It seems that seminal fluid contains prostaglandins (a chemical substance that's also made in the lining of the uterus) that cause uterine contractions. In fact, back in the old days when you had menstrual cramps, the medicine you took to control them contained an antiprostaglandin.

6. Eat "the salad." Most of you preggos have heard about "the salad" by now. It's a simple salad made at a Studio City, California, restaurant called "Caiote." It's dressed with balsamic vinaigrette that's rumored to start labor. This rumor started years ago when a woman went into labor soon after eating it. A while later, another pregnant woman went into labor after she too ate the salad. The pregnancy grapevine traveled faster than a sciatic pain and soon, women around the country were having the salad sent to them by express mail.

Luckily, I live within a few miles of the place. I went there in my thirty-eighth week, anxious for labor to begin. When I walked in, I spotted two other very pregnant women eagerly chomping away on their greens. I placed my salad order and crossed my bloated little fingers in hopes of imminent labor.

When the waiter returned with my order, I asked him if it was true. Does this magical salad actually induce labor? The waiter smiled and told me that there wasn't one woman who ate it who didn't start labor. I thanked him profusely and, with a wink, he was gone.

His wink made me suspicious. It took me a moment, but I realized what the waiter was actually saying: *Of course every pregnant woman went into labor . . . eventually.* He was admitting that the labor wasn't necessarily a reflection of eating the salad as much as it was a reflection of being pregnant for nine months. My hopes were shattered. But I wolfed down my salad anyway. Not because I felt that it would induce labor, but because it really was quite a tasty salad. And, as the waiter promised, I did go into labor. Exactly two weeks later.

Chapter Ten

Let the Bloody Show Begin

So, you're finally in labor! I bet you can't believe it. These nine months of pregnancy have sped by as fast as a long line at the DMV. But now they're over and you're on your way to the hospital. Some of you may have opted to deliver at home and are putting on your plastic sheets. Others may have chosen a birthing center and are about to dip into the Jacuzzi. Or maybe you're out in a field somewhere assuming the squatting position. But, since the vast majority of you will give birth in a hospital, majority rules, and that's where I'll focus my attention. Besides, that's where I delivered and the cardinal rule of writing is "Write what you know."

Just as I had an unrealistic idea of what pregnancy would be like, I was also in the dark about childbirth. I thought that I'd go to the hospital, have some ice chips and an epidural, huff and puff, and blow out my kid. I figured the most difficult part of my labor would be where to set up the video-camera. Man, was I ever naive.

I bet most have you have put together some kind of birth plan. All the books tell you to do so. I put together a rather vague one myself: to get this thing out of me with the least amount of pain, tearing, and stitches possible. But some women have planned their birth with the same attention to detail as a Martha Stewart wedding. And, as Murphy's Law goes, those are the women who will probably have the most difficult childbirth experience of all.

Only about 5 percent of patients go into the hospital, get their epidural when they want it, push a few times, and pop goes the weasel. This statistic is according to Sharron, a beloved delivery nurse with over forty years of experience. She works at a prominent Los Angeles hospital, and, like McDonalds, has served well over 40,000 customers. Sharron is the Queen of Contractions, the Prime Minister of Placentas, the Aficionado of Afterbirth. In fact, Sharron is such a popular delivery nurse, that second-time moms actually plan their inductions around her work schedule. As Sharron has requested, I won't use her last name (as with all mysterious informants, like "Deep Throat").

Sharron says that there's usually some kind of roadblock that you'll encounter during your delivery experience. She believes that the number one factor that will influence your process is your expectation. If you have a specific idea of how your labor should go and it's not being met, you'll feel angry. For instance, you may insist on an epidural, but you may not be far along enough to get one. Or you may only want a vaginal delivery, but end up needing a C-section. When things don't go according to your plan, you're faced with two options: either fight it or say, "What the hell?" And sometimes just that change of attitude will relax you enough to go with the flow.

For your birth experience *is* like a flow, the flow of a river. And no matter how much you obstruct it, the river is going to find a path to guide its way through. What you need to keep in mind is that the ultimate outcome of childbirth isn't a child born without drugs or forceps. The ultimate goal is to have a safe outcome for both you and the baby. And whatever it takes to make that happen is going to be the flow of your river.

If you have a specific birth plan in mind, you'll need to be realistic and informed. Although ignorance is bliss when it comes to the calorie content of a scone, it's not good when it comes to a distinct delivery blueprint. First off, you should know what to expect from your hospital. For instance, not all hospitals offer pain relievers at the same stage of labor. They all follow different safety guidelines and you should know what those guidelines are.

You also need to know what to expect from your doctor. You need to hear, not only what you want to hear, but everything he has to say. You'll want to know how long you'll to be expected to push before given a C-section. You'll want to know under what circumstance he feels forceps would be necessary. And you'll want to know when to expect to see him at the hospital. If you think that your doctor will be there to hold your hand through three hours of pushing, you were born about 100 years too late. Nowadays, it's common for the doctor to make an appearance just as the baby's head does.

My delivery was riddled with roadblocks. My birth canal was like Sunset Boulevard on New Year's Eve with police checkpoints everywhere. I thought these roadblocks made me an anomaly, but now I know that I was not. So, for the sake of a more realistic and informed childbirth experience, here are some things you may want to know before you deliver.

Inducing

When I started my ninth month, every week I would beg my O.B. to induce me and put me out of my misery. But it seemed that there are several conditions that must be met before you can be induced. And unfortunately, your strong desire to get the thing out of you already isn't one of them.

One way to warrant an induction is to be two weeks past your due date. After that, your uterus can become a hostile environment, and I can't say that I blame it. I'd be perturbed too if couldn't evict my wombmate.

A second way to allow for an induction is to be about three centimeters dilated. There are other factors involved like how thin your cervix is and how far your baby has moved down the birth canal, but three centimeters dilated is the general rule of thumb. This was the way I hoped to be induced, but every week my doctor would check me and I was always a few centimeters shy. It was as if I was being turned down for parole and forced to spend another week in my bodily prison.

If you need to be induced, there are several methods for your doctor to choose from. The most common method is the use of an intravenous drug called Pitocin. Pitocin is a form of oxytocin, a hormone that's produced naturally in your pituitary gland. It signals to your body that the thermometer on your Butterball has popped out, and it's ready to be taken out of the oven. When given Pitocin, your body should then start to make strong and regular contractions.

Another type of induction method is called a cervical ripening agent. There are several kinds to choose from, but they all do the same thing: they prime the cervix for delivery. The cervical agent ripens the cervix by causing it to thin and open so that Pitocin has a good chance of working.

The last of the induction methods is called an amniotomy. That's where the doctor breaks your bag of water. He'll take what looks like a long crochet hook, insert it into your vagina, and break the bag. Although it looks like a torture device, this crochet hook doesn't hurt a bit. In fact, there is no pain involved in breaking your water. The pain will come a few hours afterward, however, for when the water comes out, the strong contractions come in.

When I went in for my fortieth week appointment, I was in for a horrible disappointment. It was worse than if I had been turned down for inducement yet again. My doctor, the one I loved and adored, my puffy-fingered pillar of strength, had a heart attack the previous day. He had to go in for emergency heart surgery. He wouldn't be able to deliver my child! I couldn't believe it! How could he be so selfish?

I was introduced to my new doctor, Dr. Suáve (not his real name, just his real personality). Dr. Suáve was a goofy looking man with an English accent and an unpleasant smell. He no doubt went into obstetrics so that he could get his hands on things that he couldn't get his hands on otherwise. During my exam, Dr. Suáve told me that my baby was getting too big. He said that if we don't get it out soon, we were headed for a cesarean delivery. I was still only one centimeter dilated, but I wasn't about to argue with the man who was going to set me free.

Dr. Suáve suggested that I go to the hospital and he'd try to induce me. I hadn't been this happy about my pregnancy since I saw the two lines on my test. I went to the hospital and Dr. Suáve inserted one of those cervical ripening agents into my cervix. My husband joined me, and for two hours, we watched the fetal monitor in hopes that my molehill-sized contractions would turn into mountains. My husband couldn't take his eyes off the monitor. You'd think they were playing porn on the thing. I didn't realize it until that moment, but he was just as exited about me starting labor as I was. Perhaps not so much to put an end to my pregnancy as to put an end to the bloated, cranky, gassy, tired version of his wife.

But after two hours of watching my contractions (or *Debbie Does Dallas*, I'm still not sure), I was told that the goop didn't work. Mentally deflated, yet still physically inflated, I went home. But within an hour my contractions intensified. Suddenly, I became a prairie woman, lying in bed, clutching onto the headboard and screaming in pain for dear life. My husband and I raced to the hospital! There was no doubt that labor had begun.

"Lookie Loos"

Our culture exhibits some unusual behavior. We explode colorful lights in the air on the fourth day of July. We eat canned cranberries the last Thursday of November. And we turn the private act of childbirth into a family spectator sport. In other cultures, even the father of the baby isn't allowed to see its descent into the world.

It wasn't long ago that there were no visitors allowed in the delivery room. When my mom had me, they gave her an enema and a close shave (don't worry, they don't do either of those anymore) and left her alone with a Bible to read. The only way she could have someone with her was if she had taken her mother's advice and married a doctor.

But nowadays, we allow anyone who has a strong desire and an even stronger stomach to be in the room. And although these onlookers do at times provide emotional support, there are some negative aspects to having a room full of "lookie loos":

1. Sometimes, you may feel pressure when making up the delivery room guest list. Even though you may not want your mother-in-law in the room, you feel like you have to invite her since *your* mother is coming.

Miss Manners has yet to do a handbook on this topic and there are no specific etiquette guidelines to follow.

2. What do you do if your father wants to be in the room? You don't want to hurt his feelings, but you may not feel comfortable with him looking at your vagina. I know you don't feel like your body is yours anyway, but you don't want to think of the man looking at anyone's vagina . . . even your mother's.

3. Oftentimes, you don't realize what will stay in the memories of your guests. You may think they'll take with them the gift of watching your child be born, but all they'll talk about afterward is how you cut one during a really big push.

4. Sometimes, a lot of spectators can be dangerous. They tend to get in the way and obstruct the flow of safe patient care (especially during a C-section). Also, after the baby is born, the room looks more like a crime scene than a delivery room, and the hospitals, as well as OSHA, have strict policies about people tracking bodily fluids down the hallways.

Because of these scenarios, I offer some advice. First of all, talk to your nurse if you're feeling uncomfortable with any or all of the visitors. She's been through this many times and will probably know how to clear a room as fast as a bad smell. She might mention hospital policies about the number of people allowed in the room. Or she may say you need some tests that should be performed in private. Or maybe she'll just yell like a banshee that everyone leaves *now*! No matter how she'll do it, she'll clear the room fast, and we hope, without creating any ill feelings toward you.

Make sure that you tell your guests ahead of time that it's

okay if they choose to leave once you start pushing. Childbirth isn't always pretty and they should feel comfortable to leave if they want to. Your family and friends will be of no use to you or the doctors, and may even get in the way, if they stay against their better judgment.

If you want someone with you to hold your hand but don't feel comfortable with them seeing any other part of your anatomy, have them sit at the head of the table. You can drape yourself to censor the view and still get the head rub you so deserve.

If you intend to take pictures, either photographs or videotape, make sure to clear it with the hospital staff first. Most of them won't mind since they've been photographed more than Hugh Grant after the hooker incident. But others may be more like Sean Penn and want to punch your lights out if you point and click.

How to Breathe Through a Contraction

I bet you thought somewhere during your pregnancy how great it was not to get your period. No cramps for a whole nine months! Well, now it's payback time! For one contraction is like nine months' worth of cramps rolled up into one big achy ball.

There are no words to describe the pain of a contraction. I guess it would be somewhat like digging your eyeball out with a blunt nail. And I mean a rusty one to boot. I'm not talking about the early contractions where you can still carry on a conversation. I'm talking about the hard core ones that make you fall to the floor.

When I got to the hospital, I was examined by Nurse Satan (not her real name, just her nearest relative). I begged her for some pain medicine, but she said that I was only one

“ After a couple of hours of labor my doctor came to my room. I was so happy to see him and I told him I was ready to get this baby out now. He said the baby's not going anywhere until that smile was wiped off my face. **”**

—My grandma Sally

centimeter dilated. She couldn't even admit me into the hospital yet, let alone give me something for the pain. She told me to walk around for an hour and she'd check me again.

I spent the next hour in contraction hell and I brought my husband along for the ride. Every time a contraction hit, I would grab him by some part of his anatomy and scream. I had my long pregnancy nails and wasn't afraid to use them. I knew that I was hurting him, but it was only fair that he experience a fraction of the pain that I was in.

After an eternity, the hour passed. As promised Nurse Satan re-examined me and, to her surprise, found that I was now at four centimeters. Normally, it takes about four hours to go from one to four centimeters during active labor, so she knew things were happening quickly. She finally checked me into the hospital and gave me a shot for the pain.

This is exactly what I was telling you about, that hospitals have their own set of guidelines to follow. And although I hated Nurse Satan at the time for not checking me in and giving me medicine, she did have her reasons. For one, most hospitals and insurance companies allow for a two-day stay for vaginal deliveries. If a patient is admitted too early, there could be a shortage of beds and maybe even an increase in the amount of the patient's bill. Also, an epidural can slow labor if given too early.

If you're far enough along, you'll be checked in and given

drugs to help with the pain. But if you're still in the early stages of labor, or if you just don't want drugs at all, there is one thing you can do to control the pain of a contraction: Breathe. I guarantee that if you fight the pain, or feed into it, it will become much worse. I know that I did this many times. I would feel a contraction start and I was so afraid, I would clench up and panic. But if you can catch the pain early on, and breathe with it, you'll have an easier time than if you didn't breathe at all. I don't want to mislead you. Even with proper breathing, there will still be pain. But it will be more controlled.

There are several different breathing techniques, from short, fast breaths to long and slow ones, but the one that Nurse Sharron recommends to her patients is to breathe in slowly for a count of five, hold it for a second or two, then release it for another slow count of five. You should think of this breathing as the gentle rhythmic laps of the ocean. The key to its success is that you start breathing the instant that you feel the contraction coming on. If you miss it, you can't play catch-up.

You can try many different techniques while you breathe. Try them all or think of some of your own. Just do whatever feels the most comfortable for you.

1. Put your arms around your significant other's shoulders and put your head into his chest. Round your pelvis and rock as you breathe. If it feels good, your partner can rub your lower back at the same time.
2. Go down on all fours, again with a rounded back. Breathe and rock through the pain.
3. If you're at home, or if your hospital is equipped with one, take a warm shower. Some women find this to be very soothing.

4. Sit on a big rubber exercise ball. There's something wonderful about the way your perineum fits on top if it. It's pliable on your joints as well. Not all hospitals have them, so you may have to bring your own. You can find them at sporting good stores and those that sell exercise equipment.

5. Lie down on the cold floor. This was my personal favorite. The shock of the coldness distracted me from the pain going on underneath my skin. You can't do this in the later stages of labor since you'll need to be hooked up to a fetal monitor.

6. Have a hard foot massage.

7. Use a labor doula. A doula is a support person trained in the field of labor. Again, you have to bring your own, and I recommend that you find one who's well recommended. Just like any professional, there are incredible ones and iffy ones.

Gimme Drugs

For me, drugs are as important to childbirth as raisins are to rice pudding. But many women disagree (not about the pudding thing). They want to experience childbirth naturally. And although I applaud their determination, I'm confused by their logic. It'd be like going to the dentist for root canal and asking her not to give you any Novocain.

When it comes to drugs, there are several different ones to choose from. Most all hospitals are equipped with the grandmama of them all, the epidural, but there are other drugs available as well. Each hospital has their preferences, so it's important to check with them beforehand if you have a specific painkiller in mind. My hospital was a fan of fentanyl. And, although it didn't take the pain away, it did take enough of the edge off so that I could get up from the cold hard floor.

Although the painkiller helped, I told Nurse Satan that I wanted an epidural too. I was under the illusion, or should I say delusion, that there was an anesthesiologist waiting outside my door to administer my drugs whenever I felt the urge. But that's rarely the case.

Some hospitals don't have a dedicated anesthesiologist on the floor. Sometimes, they can be tied up in another ward with another patient, or maybe in an emergency C-section. And even if there is one on the floor, it's not like they walk in and give you a shot. First, they have to take a history, interview and assess you, tell you what you can expect and not expect, and inform you what's available from their product line. They're like the Mary Kay girls of anesthesia.

Nurse Satan told me that I should get the epidural in about half an hour. She also told me that my doctor was on the way. I was so happy. I wasn't going home, I was going to have a baby, and better still, I was going to have an epidural! All I had to do was hold out for thirty more minutes and I would be free of pain. I could do this; I could hold on!

As promised, after a half an hour of screaming in pain (by both me and my husband), the door opened. But it was not the anesthesiologist as I had hoped. It was Dr. Suáve strolling in wearing his workout attire. I obviously disturbed him at the gym where he was exercising his retinas staring at women on the inner thigh machine.

He gave me an internal exam and announced, with amazement, that I was at ten centimeters. It was time to push! I had gone from four to ten centimeters in half an hour. I became an honorary graduate of the Evelyn Wood speed dilation school.

I told him that I couldn't stand the pain for one more second and to *please* give me my epidural now. But then Dr. Suáve uttered the most horrible words that I've ever heard. He told me that I couldn't have an epidural. It was too late. He said that an epidural is impossible for a patient who's fully dilated. My husband looked at the welts in his arms and begged the doctor to change his mind. Dr. Suáve told us that I had to be able to feel the contractions so that I'd know when to push. Oh, it was time to push all right. It was time to push him right out the window!

I don't mean to scare you. Unless you're a speed dilator too, there should be ample time for you to get an epidural. You will probably be spared the horrible pain that only child-birth or a bad tractor accident can cause. For the most part epidurals are quite safe with very few side effects, but there are some things that you should know about:

1. In a very small percentage of women, the numbness created by an epidural goes up too high and you can get a sense that you can't breathe. Although it's scary, you *can* still breathe and are never in danger.
2. Just like with Demerol, an epidural can cause nausea.
3. Sometimes, it feels as if you lose control of your legs. You think you're so numb that you can't move them, but you can.
4. There's a big misnomer about epidurals. You think that if you're given one, you're not going to feel anything. But that's not true. The key to a successful epidural is to be pain free, not sensation free. You want to be able to push when they need you to push. And even though you won't feel the intense pain, you will still feel the pressure of the baby, and that can be quite uncomfortable in itself.

5. As with any drug, you may find that you're allergic to it at an inopportune time. You may develop hives or a rash. Unfortunately, this can't be prevented.

6. Occasionally, an epidural may cause some mild but uncontrollable shaking. This is less due to the epidural than the additional IV fluids that will need to be administered.

7. If your grandma is with you, an epidural may cause her to cry. She'll be so jealous that she'll rant and rave about her childbirth stories, and about how the only painkiller she had was her tongue to bite on. These tales can be more painful than labor.

How to Push with a Passion

Believe it or not, you could deliver your baby without pushing at all. Women in comas do it all the time. Sure, it may take a week or two, but eventually the baby comes out. There are many factors that determine how long it takes to push out your kid. Sometimes, it takes just a few pushes. Other times, it could take several hours' worth.

You'll obviously have a tougher time if your baby's head is large, or if your pelvic bones are narrow. It'll also take longer if your baby hasn't descended far down the birth canal by the time you're ready to push. Sometimes, one woman can be a better pusher than another one, not because she's been working out at a better gym, but because she's pushing more effectively, for there is a right way and a wrong way to push.

One of the biggest no-no's to do when you push is to scream. Although screaming is fine when you're making the baby, it's not fine to do when you're trying to get it out of you. If you scream it means that you're not holding your breath, and you need to hold your breath to push effectively.

Another no-no is to push from your chest. This is a complete waste of energy and very ineffective. What you need to do is to push from farther down your body. Although most of you have heard that you should push as if you're having a bowel movement, Nurse Sharron doesn't agree. She feels that pushing out a baby is more like peeing than pooping.

For the past few months, you've had to pee so often, that you've learned to squeeze every bit of urine out of your bladder so you won't have to go to the bathroom again so quickly. Pushing out a baby is similar to that. The muscles that are used to pushing out that last drop of urine are the same ones that make for the most productive pushing. If you try to think of it like that, you'll connect with the right mechanism used to push effectively.

There are different positions you can use while you push, and it's important to find one that works best for you. One of the most difficult, yet important aspects of effective pushing is to not lose your stamina while you're doing it. If exhaustion sets in, you won't have the strength to keep at it for a long period of time. I've listed some of the more popular pushing positions. Some will feel better than others, so try to find one that works best for you. Mix and match if you like, or ask your nurse if she has any other ideas.

1. Sit straight up like on a toilet.
2. Have the head of your bed raised so that your torso is at about a forty-five degree angle to your legs.
3. Lie flat on your back with your legs up so that your knees are near your ears.

4. While lying down, put your hands underneath your thighs while keeping your elbows out.

5. Hold onto your bed handles (if they're available at your hospital). They're movable, so find a position that works best for you.

6. Put your feet up in the stirrups.

7. Squat using a squatting bar (if there is one). This position may take some coordination, but it's quite popular as it's the age-old way to deliver a baby.

Nurse Satan didn't give me much choice about my pushing position and I didn't know that I had any to choose from. She lay me down on my back and put my legs up high. She then stood next to me and pushed down on my stomach during each contraction like she was trying to move a stalled car. After two hours of this, Dr. Suáve came in. He was worried and said if I couldn't get my baby out soon, I would need a cesarean. There it was—the dreaded "C" word. The mere thought of it threw my pushing power into high gear. I'm surprised my daughter didn't pop out of me like a champagne cork.

He told me we'd make one last-ditch effort to get her out before he cut her out. It was then that he called in "the Vacuum." They wheeled in a big machine that had a plunger-like cup on one end. He stuck the cup inside me and attached it to the crown of my baby's head. They were going to suck out my baby like a bad clog!

After a few moments of plunging, her head finally popped out. It worked! I wasn't going to need a C-section after all. Dr. Suáve asked me if I wanted to take a look at my baby's head, and without a second thought, I declined. For I knew that the eight seconds that it would take for me to lift up my head, take a peek, and put my head back down on the pillow would be enough time for one more contraction to set in. That, in a nutshell, was how bad the pain was. It was so unbearable that I passed on seeing my child emerge into the world.

After one more painful push, my baby squished out of me like toothpaste from a tube. She was an absolutely beautiful baby, with adorable features and in perfect health. I couldn't have been happier, although I guess my expectations were pretty low. All I wanted was a child with skin. By the way, my gigantic baby weighed in at only 6 pounds, 12 ounces. Any other doctor could have taken her out with a pair of tweezers.

Episiotomy: Let 'er Rip

An episiotomy is a procedure where the doctor makes an incision at the back of your vagina in order to give the baby more room to get out. It sounds like a horrible thing and I can't help but feel that it's man's revenge for the invention of the circumcision. Many people, especially midwives, feel that episiotomies are unnecessary in any situation.

Most doctors do try to avoid them. They massage and stretch the perineum using mineral oil. They hope that this will lubricate the tissue, decreasing its resistance so that it will stretch out. But, if that doesn't work, the doctor has a decision about an incision.

Just by looking at the crowning baby, the doctor can get a good idea of the baby's size. If the head appears small, he may choose to let the baby make a small tear on its own when it pushes through. But, if the doctor feels that the baby's head is big, and a large uncontrolled tear is probable, he'll no doubt do an episiotomy. If this is the case, he'll inject the area with a numbing agent and make an incision to allow for more room.

There are four different degrees of a tear that the baby

can inflict. The first degree is the least severe. It's a small tear that will require just a few stitches for the repair. The fourth degree, however, is pretty intense since the tear goes past your anus. The repair process is much more intricate. It will take about twenty to thirty minutes to repair and may need as many stitches as a Vera Wang gown.

I know that the thought of having a knife slice through your genitals sounds horrid, but I promise, it will seem insignificant with everything that's going on around you. What with the nausea and the unimaginable pain of the contractions, an episiotomy is like a mere paper cut in your day.

The "C" Word

For many women, a cesarean section comes as no surprise. For numerous reasons—for instance, if you have a condition like previa or diabetes—it may have been scheduled far in advance. But for other women, a C-section comes out of left field. A woman can endure hours of labor and then something goes wrong. When she's told that a C-section is necessary, it can be very upsetting. She may feel as if she's failed. She may feel horribly guilty. Or she may just feel terrified of going under the knife. For even though a C-section may be the safer way to deliver the baby, it still means that she'll be pried open like a can of sardines.

There are various reasons that a C-section may become necessary. Here are some common case scenarios:

1. You're dilated to ten centimeters and have pushed for two or three hours, but for some reason, the baby just isn't coming out. Maybe the baby is too big or it's in the wrong position. Your doctor may have tried the vacuum or maybe even forceps, but still no baby.

2. The baby is in distress. Although delivery is stressful on you, it also takes its toll on your child. The medical staff watches the baby's fetal monitor for any sign of distress, and if any show up, it may need to come out in less time than a vaginal delivery could take.

3. The baby is in the breech position. This doesn't happen very often, but if it's determined that a baby is breech, it will almost always be delivered with a C-section (see Don't Breech to Me on page 155).

4. Your cervix has stopped dilating. If a cervix gets stuck, it usually happens between five and seven centimeters. Your doctor will try to break your water and use pitocin, but if it still refuses to dilate any further, it's C-section city for you.

If you need a C-section, you're hooked up to an IV and given either an epidural or a spinal (a spinal blocks all feeling). Your pubic hair will be shaved so you don't get hair in the incision. Your bladder will be emptied using a catheter so your doctor won't mistake your ballooning bladder for your baby's head. The physician will then test your skin for numbness and wash your belly with an antiseptic solution He'll put sterile drapes in front of you so you can't see what's going on, and make an incision right below your bikini line. In anywhere from five to twenty minutes, your star is born!

Most women are under the impression that they won't feel anything during a cesarean delivery, but that's not true. For one thing, the drugs may make you feel nauseated and may even make you feel as if you're going through a tunnel. Both of these sensations are caused by the painkillers and are treatable. Also, if you have an epidural, you'll still feel pressure as the doctor tries to get the baby out. It may take some manipulation, especially if your baby has descended far down your vagina. Some women feel as if the air is being knocked out of them.

I know that a C-section may sound scary, but there are benefits to having one. You won't need an episiotomy, and your perineum stays more or less intact so you'll have less pain with postpartum sex and pooping. And, if your C-section is scheduled, you can squeeze in childbirth after you've picked up your dry-cleaning. You also won't have to endure a painful labor, and you'll have some control over your child's birthday. With vaginal deliveries, your baby could share the same birthday with Hitler and there's not a damn thing you can do about it.

Bonding

I think bonding is yet another big lie of reproduction. Although sometimes women can hear harps playing in the background when their baby arrives, other times it can be very anticlimactic. And when this happens, it makes the new mother feel as if there's something wrong with her.

If you don't bond with your child the first time you see it, don't worry. This is actually a more common occurrence than you think. For one thing, you've just endured hours of grueling labor. You're exhausted and weak. The only thing you want to hold is a hotel room key for a few days of R&R. For another, the nurse usually hands you your baby while the doctor is busy pulling out your placenta, or sewing up a tear. This may not be the proper ambiance for a Kodak moment.

Sure, you've seen movies and television shows of births, and may have witnessed firsthand the joy that bringing a newborn baby into this world can bring to its new mother. But maybe, just maybe, her tears of happiness and blazing smile are a result of her realizing that her contractions are over and that she's no longer pregnant.

Sometimes, mothers can be taken back by the appearance of their child. They may have thought that all newborns look like Ivory Snow babies, when the truth is that they don't. Some have cone heads from being squeezed through a tight birth canal. Others may be bald or have a thick pelt of hair. Oftentimes, their eyes are puffy and their skin is blotchy. They could also have hair covering their back, shoulders, and forehead. Your baby may look more like a member of the Lollipop Guild than a member of your own family.

I wish I could tell you that when my daughter was born it was a magical moment. That seeing her for the first time brought tears to my eyes, and made me realize the essence of womanhood. But the truth is that I was so exhausted from pushing that it took every ounce of energy I had just to blink. I was hesitant to touch her at first. As with all newborns, she was covered with a slimy substance that made her look like a giant piece of gefilte fish.

But eventually I did bond with my daughter. It didn't happen right away; in fact, it took several days. But once it set in, it set in hard, and I couldn't imagine loving anyone more. So, if you don't bond with your child in an instant, give yourself a break and a couple of days. I promise it will happen.

What to Do When Nature Calls

The baby was out! The baby was out! Hi ho, the baby was out! As excited as I was to see my baby's precious face on the outside of my inside, I was just as excited, if not more, that my pregnancy was over. That night in the hospital, I slept on my stomach for the first time in months. I didn't take an antacid for the first time in months. And even though I was still grossly overweight, I had never felt so skinny in my life.

But it wasn't all fun. There is a reason that a woman must stay in the hospital after she delivers. She needs time to heal. She needs around-the-clock nursing care. She needs strong pain medication.

I stayed in the hospital for two days. I had wonderful nurses who took care of me. They put ice packs on my privates and helped me figure out how to breastfeed. They brought me tasty meals and changed my dirty sheets. But, as much as I wished that they could, there was one thing that they couldn't do for me. There was one thing I had to do on my own. That thing was going to the bathroom.

Number One

It won't be long after you deliver that you'll feel the urge to pee. What with your IV fluids and your excess bodily ones, it's only a matter of time until your bladder is full. For me it happened in just a couple of hours. I tried to hold it in as long as I could. The thought of peeing all over the fresh stitches terrified me. But I couldn't hold it in any longer and hobbled to the bathroom.

I looked at the toilet as if it were a medieval torture device. What was once a private sanctuary had now become hostile territory. I had to be brave like my foremothers before me. So I lowered my achy, pain-ridden body down onto the seat, took a deep breath, and went for it. And you know what? It didn't hurt at all. Not one little bit.

But the act of peeing was no simple matter anymore. This basic bodily function entailed more steps than the Empire State Building. Every time I went to the bathroom, there was a list of procedures that I had to go through. After I peed,

I had to carefully blot myself dry. They I sprayed myself with an antiseptic spray. This spray was a great invention. It was cooling and numbing, and eased the pain. After the spray came the witch hazel pads that had to be carefully applied to the stitches. Then I had to change sanitary pads to deal with all the blood (more on that later). This process of blot/spray/ wipe/change would take so long that by the time I finished with my bathroom ritual, I had to pee again.

When nature calls, I have some suggestions to help deal with postpartum peeing:

1. The first time that you need to go to the bathroom after you deliver, take a nurse with you. They'll provide a wash bottle and all the other accoutrements necessary to excrete.

2. You may feel a very slight burn, and if you do, it will only happen that one time.

3. Make sure that you bring all the bottles and sprays home with you from the hospital. While you're at it, take the sanitary napkins, nasal aspirator, gauze pads, diapers, water bottles, and nipples as well. The truth is that you're going to be billed for that stuff anyway, so you may as well take it all with you. It's the equivalent of the tiny soap and shampoo bottles in hotel bathrooms.

4. At home you should have a bottle of witch hazel in your refrigerator. Pour some on a nonmedicated makeup pad remover and apply it to your wounds. The coldness of the witch hazel will feel quite soothing.

Number Two

Unlike going number one, number two is no easy feat after childbirth. In fact, it can be quite traumatic. Ask any

"I had a fourth degree tear and it'd been sixteen days since I pooped. When I couldn't hold it in any longer, I made my husband race home from work to watch our son. Although I finally went, my husband lost a sale. That poop cost us five hundred dollars in commission.**"**

—Kelly

mother about her first poop after delivery and her eyes will glaze over like a holiday ham. She'll tremble and sweat as the memory of this terrifying event comes flooding back. This woman is experiencing post-traumatic stress disorder, not unlike veterans who relive the horrors of war.

If you had an epidural, this kind of "delivery" may be more painful than pushing out your kid. Understandably, the perineal area is very sore from the bruises, swelling, and possible hemorrhoids. And if you had an episiotomy, you'll be convinced that you're going to blow out the stitches with the very first push. For me, the event was so painful, I felt as if I were pushing out an undetected twin.

But fret not, there are some ways to make your daily doodee a little less difficult:

1. Take a stool softener. If I can teach you one thing in this book, it's the importance of a good stool softener. You'll probably be given one in the hospital, but if you're not, ask for one! Beg for one! And make sure that you continue to use them at home.
2. Take a pain reliever about an hour before you attempt to poop. If you're at home, try ibuprofen. This should help with any pain, and knowing this may help you relax a bit.
3. Drink something hot each morning to help stimulate pooping contractions.

4. Make sure that your diet is high in fiber.

5. Use a padded toilet seat cover. I found that sitting on the toilet for any longer than ten seconds made me cry. It put strain on parts of me that I didn't want to strain ever again. I didn't have a padded toilet seat so I lined my toilet with a towel. You can try this in a pinch.

6. Don't worry about ripping out your stitches. The main reason for the mental anguish is that you'll be afraid that the pushing will tear you open. But I promise it won't. The string they use to tie you back together with could be used as elevator cable. It ain't going nowhere.

Even with all these precautions, you may still have some discomfort. I wish I could tell you that after the first poop is over, everything will be okay. But it's not. It will be better though. You'll realize that you won't rip your stitches out and you'll discover that the buildup is, as usual, worse than the actual event.

I promise that it gets easier with every poop and that things will return to normal in a couple of weeks. You'll go to the bathroom without even thinking about it just like in the good old days. You may even bring some reading material in there with you as well. But unlike the old days, you now have a newborn and won't have time to read for eighteen more years.

Lochia: Who Knew?

After my baby was born, I thought I was done with things coming out of my vagina for a while. But wrong I was. In fact, after a baby is born there's a great deal of blood that will flow for a great deal of time. This flow is called lochia and it's made up of extra blood, tissue, and mucus that's being excreted from your uterus. The flow is rather heavy for the first several days so you'll need to have plenty of sanitary pads available. For the first few days, I wore two at a time and bled through both in a matter of hours.

The amount of blood will dissipate as the days go by. What was once as mighty as Niagara Falls will soon become a trickle. This is where that disposable underwear will get its last hurrah. By the fifth week, my bleeding stopped completely and everything was back to normal. In fact, I didn't have any more vaginal bleeding for eight whole months when I finally got a period. That alone should be worth the horrors of delivery.

In addition to the flow being heavy and lengthy, it's also quite colorful. At first the blood is red, but after a while it turns to a soft shade of pink, then brown, yellow, and finally, eggshell. A lochia bleed is like a beautiful vaginal rainbow.

Got Milk?

Within minutes of being born, your baby will want to eat. This surprised me at first. I mean, the kid ate through its umbilical cord that was cut just moments ago, and already it's chow time? How did she get so hungry? It's not like she had to reshingle a roof on her way down the canal.

But, being a good mom, I put my hungry kid to my breast and she, being a good kid, started sucking away. I wasn't sure that there was anything in me to suck. In the last weeks of pregnancy I thought that I'd leak some colostrum, but I never did. I guess there was some kind of nutrient in me because several hours after she nursed, she was still alive.

I hear that breastfeeding can be a frustrating and painful

experience, but I was very lucky. For one thing, my daughter was a natural-born breastfeeder and would latch on like a tick. For another, I had a body for feeding. As I've told you before, my breasts were enormous. I had enough room in there for a gallon of milk, plus a dozen eggs and some cheese. I think that when I go back to work, I'm going become a wet nurse. I shouldn't let these boobs go to waste. There are plenty of poor starving preschoolers all over the world.

Not all women have an easy time of it. Many say that it's very painful when the baby nurses. Their nipples crack and their breasts would clog and engorgement was always a problem. For them, breastfeeding is a miserable event.

I hope that you have an easy time of it. If you don't, there are many support groups to turn to. Ask your doctor, the hospital, or your pediatrician for some references. These groups are full of advice for common ailments like sore nipples and pumping problems. In addition to their advice, I'd like to provide some of my own:

1. The most important trick to breastfeeding is to make sure that your child latches on properly. It's crucial that she open her mouth wide enough to take in more than just your nipple. As soon as your baby's mouth is open *really* wide, slap her on you quickly before she has a chance to close her mouth.

2. Stock up on lanolin. It's great to use on sore nipples and it won't harm your baby.

3. Put together a nursing kit. Whenever I fed my daughter, it was just a matter of time before I needed something. So I filled a basket with the television remote, the telephone, a glass of water (nursing made me thirsty), and some goodies (it also made me hungry).

4. If you find yourself with a tender lump in your breast,

or your breasts become severely sore, hard, red or swollen, you may have either a breast clog or a breast infection. In either case, you should ask your doctor or lactation specialist for advice.

If, either at the hospital or after you've tried breastfeeding, you decide that nursing isn't for you, you'll have to go through the physical pain of engorgement while your body stops producing milk. This means hard, leaky, swollen, and painful breasts. In addition to the physical problems, you may also have some emotional concerns as well. For today, there is so much pressure from society and health care providers to breastfeed your newborn that you may feel guilty about your decision to stop.

Personally, I feel that it's unjust. Having a newborn is stressful enough without having to deal with leaky breasts and bloody nipples. Sure, breast milk is best, but formula is very nutritious, and as long as you're not feeding your child Kool-Aid, your baby should be just fine. My mother never breastfed me and I turned out all right. I never got sick much and I have rather good teeth. So, just stick to your guns. You know what's best for both you and your baby. You're a mother now and mothers are always right, right? Besides, having bottles around can be quite useful. They're ideal for mixing salad dressing in because the measurements along the side allow for the perfect oil to vinegar ratio.

Chapter Eleven

Home, Bittersweet Home

I know some of you might be thinking, "Hey, the pregnancy part is over. I've endured these past nine months and now the hard part is over. Why are there still so many pages of the book left?" Yes, I know that you're no longer pregnant, but for some, the hard part is not over. And I feel that it's my obligation to inform some of you how difficult your life may become with your new home addition. Don't worry. These extra pages won't cost you a thing. This book would be priced the same with or without this bonus chapter. I simply feel it's my public duty to inform you of something. For as much as pregnancy may have sucked, having a newborn can, at times, be pretty sucky as well.

This won't be the case for all of you. Some of you will have been blessed with a baby who's a good sleeper and only cries when it's hungry. But some of you may not have been, and this chapter is for you.

My child was a crier. Every evening, without fail, she'd cry for two hours straight. She was also a light sleeper who needed twenty minutes of absolute silence in order to fall into a deep sleep. During that time, we couldn't walk around the house because the hardwood floors might creak. We couldn't turn on a light switch on the other side of the house for fear that the "click" would wake her up. Thank God the space shuttle wasn't in orbit or she'd have been up all night.

She was also very high maintenance. She was only happy if I walked her around in my arms while bouncing her up and down at the same time. If I sat down for a moment she'd start to scream. I couldn't leave her in one place for more than five minutes without her getting bored. I'd have to rotate her like a tire from one activity to the next.

From the moment you step over the threshold with your child, a cosmic shift takes place in the universe. Before this moment, everything was centered around you. "How are you feeling?" "Let me carry your bag for you." "Here, take my seat." But now that the baby's out, that's all history.

Here I was, just home from the hospital, feeling like the most sensitive part of my body was put through a paper shredder. I wasn't able to sit or stand and no one seemed to care. Even my mother, who normally wanted to take care of me if I had a hunger pang, didn't care. She pretended to. She'd bring me water or talk to me from time to time. But she was too excited about her first grandchild to be very convincing. It was then that I understood how ignored my husband must have felt during these past nine months.

I learned many things when my baby was a newborn. Like pregnancy, there always seems to be a hurdle to overcome and, once you did, there was another one butted up right smack against it. Because of this, I want to pass along some tips. They may make your life just a little bit easier, or they may do nothing at all. But even if they do nothing the first time you try them, I've learned one thing about parenting. Kids go through stages and go through them quickly.

While you wait, when a problem arises—and it will—try different things to solve it. Use your common sense and a little imagination. Put yourself in your baby's head in hopes of understanding his point of view. And if that doesn't work, stick a pacifier in his mouth and call it a day.

Baby Blues

Although there were moments of utter contentment and bliss after I had my baby, there were others that were so bad I wondered why I ever wanted a child in the first place. I had just spent the past three hours trying to get my child to sleep only to have the phone wake her up. I was so sick of never being able to take a bite of food without being interrupted, and never having a minute to call my own. I hadn't spent one quality moment with my husband in months and couldn't find time to pay the bills or return phone calls. I missed my old life and wondered if things would ever settle down.

At first, I was too embarrassed to admit how I felt to anyone. If someone called to ask how things were going, I gave them the obligatory "Everything's great. I've never been happier in my life," response. It was too scary to admit how I was really feeling. Too ashamed to say that, at times, I was miserable and felt trapped. I couldn't even say those things to my husband. What would he think of me?

But finally, there came a time when I could hold it in no more. I got a call from my friend Lisa. I had slept a total of two hours the night before, and spent the morning walking my crying child around the house until I had blisters on my feet. I didn't have time for that desperately needed cup of coffee, let alone to get dressed or take a shower. No matter how hard I tried, I could not get my daughter to sleep.

So, when I heard Lisa's voice on the other end of the

phone, I crumbled. I tried to hold back the tears as I said aloud the words I swore I would never say: "I hate this." I told her. "I had no idea motherhood would be this hard, and (*gulp*) a part of me wishes that I never had a child."

But instead of telling me that she was going to call Social Services, Lisa told me that she felt the same way after her daughter was born. She told me about her breakdowns and how her colicky baby needed to be driven around the neighborhood all night to get any sleep. And about how stressful it was on her marriage, and that she too started to resent her child. Then she told me the words that I desperately longed to hear. She said that, at some point, every new mother she knew felt the same way that I did.

Lisa promised that things would get better. She said that something happens when your baby is three months old that turns things around. She said that things get even better at six months and from then on it's much more manageable. She said that if it didn't, she wouldn't be doing what she's doing. And then she told me her something she had yet to tell her husband: that she was pregnant again.

I guess that was the proof that I was looking for. Those were the magic words that made me believe that I could really pull this off. If motherhood was really that bad, people wouldn't possibly be so stupid as to have more than one kid.

I was thrilled. It turns out that I wasn't the worst mother in the world. I was just a new mother. I now worship Lisa and call her my hero. She got me through one of the most difficult stretches of this whole childrearing process, and for that I would do anything for her. Even babysit her future newborn . . . for an hour or so.

For those of you who are struggling with these first few months, try to get some support. Call friends who have young kids. Join "mommy and me" groups. Go to the parks. Go to the food courts at the malls. It's not hard to find new mothers and once you find them, you'll bond as fast as quick-drying cement. New mothers need each other desperately. They're an excellent source of support and can make the difference between tears of sorrow and tears of joy.

In addition, it's crucial that you get away from your baby from time to time. One of the best ways to handle your new responsibility is to flee from it. Even a half hour alone in the park can do wonders when you don't have the weight of your infant, its carrier, its diaper bag, and a U-Haul's worth of baby paraphernalia on your shoulders. If you have a close friend or family member to watch your baby, ask him or her. If not, hire a responsible sitter. It may cost money, but it's a lot cheaper than the therapy bills from having a mental breakdown.

How to Deal with Visitors

Nothing fills a home with visitors more than a new baby. You may as well have swaddled up Tom Cruise and brought him home in your infant carrier. All you want is to be left alone with your baby and rest up after delivery. But every friend, family member, neighbor, and gas meter reader within a forty-mile radius wants to check out the new "celebrity." Your phone will ring off the hook with friends who want to schedule viewings. They'll come over at all hours of the day and night, and some will just drop by unannounced.

With few exceptions, these visitors don't just take a quick peek and leave. For some reason, they feel that driving over with a gift in hand entitles them to stay for long periods of time. They expect to hold the baby whether it's asleep or awake. They expect elaborate stories about your delivery. Worse yet, they expect food.

I was never in the mood for visitors. Somehow the idea of assembling an hors d'oeuvre tray never appealed to me when my privates were just lanced like a boil. I know these visitors mean well, but they can be very thoughtless. Maybe they forget how overwhelming it is to have a little creature invade your home. Or maybe they're bad at picking up on clues like "I could really use a good nap about now." Either way, I suggest the following to keep you sane, or some resemblance thereof:

1. **Don't answer the phone.** If there's ever a time to screen your calls, this is it. Our problem was that the phone machine was in our bedroom along with the bassinet, so often we were forced to answer the phone for fear the machine would wake our daughter up. If this is your situation, rewire the house immediately.

2. **Invite only those family members you truly want to see and let the other ones slide for now.** I know this sounds mean and selfish, but you just gave life to a baby, and you only have so much to give.

3. **The only exception to rule number two is that even if you don't like them, accept visitors from anyone who offers to bring you food.** I would have had Leona Helmsley over if she brought along a bucket of chicken. Food, especially that which is pre-cooked, will become more valuable to you than gold.

4. **Get used to saying "No."** People are going to invite themselves over and now is the time to use your backbone. And your husband better develop one, too. Whenever mine answered the phone, he agreed to a visit. I would tell him that I didn't want to see anyone who had more than a week to live. He then had to

call the person back and recant. This adds yet more stress to your already stressful life.

5. **If you do invite someone over, give him or her an out time.** Mention something like from twelve to one o'clock would be a good time for a visit because we have to be at the pediatrician's office at shortly after one.

6. **Be prepared for drop-ins.** I was astounded at the amount of people who had the nerve just to drop by unannounced whenever they wanted to see the baby. They must be under the delusion that we live in Mayberry. Of course, people would invariably come by when I was napping. To solve this problem, my husband made me a sign for the front door that read "Nap Time. Please *Call* Later." Some people got the message. Others did not. To this day, I still don't speak to the "others."

Like all things, this barrage of phone calls and visitors won't last forever. It took about two weeks before the number of calls started to decrease. And then, after a few more weeks, they stopped completely. No more calls. No more visitors. No more anything. I figure that most of my friends stopped calling because I never had the time to talk. The others stopped because, if I had the time to talk, they got sick of what I was talking about: the baby. I used to have friends. Now I have a newborn.

I figure that in time things will get back to normal. I'll come home and there will be a message on the machine. Someone may even invite us over for a barbecue. But for now, my social life revolves around a "mommy and me" class and a stroll to the park for a swing ride. And that's about all the social life I can handle right about now.

Better Sleep for You and Your Baby

Getting your baby to sleep is difficult. There are entire books devoted to this subject alone. And the truth is that no one method works for all babies. Some like a quiet room, while others prefer noise. Some like vibrations, whereas others like to be rocked. Also, what works once won't always work the next time. Baby's need change from week to week, even from day to day.

Then, once you get her to sleep, you'll worry if she sleeps too long. You fear that she'll miss a feeding or she'll be up all night. You try to wake her, but it's difficult. It's as if she downed a couple of Nytols when your head was turned. And once you do wake her, she's tired and cranky, so you struggle to get her back to sleep. It seems that you spend the majority of the day either trying to wake her up or getting her back to sleep.

We had another sleeping problem that perhaps you share. Once we got our daughter asleep in our arms, she'd wake up whenever we'd lower her into the bassinet. Inevitably, her arms would flail out to her sides and all three of us would start to cry. It seems that babies are born with a startle reflex that sets off whenever they're lowered.

We tried everything we could to stop this reflex. We lowered her in feet first. We lowered her in headfirst. We lowered her in slowly, then quickly; then from one side, then the other. It was driving us crazy. But, finally, we found a solution. My neighbor suggested that we swaddle her up tight like a well-made burrito. She felt snug and secure and more often than not didn't even notice that we were lowering her into her bassinet.

Because of the flailing reflex, I think that bassinets are useless. I don't care how cute it may be, or how many generations of family members have used it before you, bassinets are poorly designed. The problem with them is that their walls are much too deep. Where do they think the kid is going anyway? It can't even lift its head, let alone scale the walls of the bassinet.

In most cases, every month your sleeping problems get easier and easier. Your baby will be able to sleep for longer stretches at a time, and that means you can too. There will actually be a day when you'll wake up in the morning before your baby does. And that will be the one of the greatest days of your life.

Baby Hygiene

For the most part, keeping your newborn clean is quite easy. There are no teeth to brush, and little or no hair to manage. Give your kid a bath from time to time and you're more or less done.

But there are two tricky areas of your baby that may need special care: The first are the fingernails. When my baby arrived, she had perfectly trimmed nails. It was as if there were a manicurist up there inside my uterus. But not long after my baby came home, her nails grew quite long quite quickly. I took out my infant nail clippers and tried to cut them, but it was difficult to get the clippers to fit underneath her itty-bitty nails. I may as well have been using garden shears.

But then it happened. As I tried to clip one of her nails, I clipped off part of her finger instead! It was just the very tippy top, but enough to cause some damage. Instantly, she started wailing as the blood dripped from her precious little finger. To make matters worse, my in-laws had just flown in for a visit and were there to witness the maiming of their granddaughter.

Although my poor infant stopped crying in only a few minutes and I got the bleeding to stop, I was traumatized. I had hurt my baby and made her cry. And because of me, my daughter was going to have the hands of a wood shop teacher.

I could never face the clippers again. Instead, I started biting her nails off. It's amazing how sensitive your mouth is and how much safer it seemed than those torturous clippers. I've been biting my nails for years and have yet to munch off the top of my own finger. If you're not comfortable with biting, try simply peeling them off. Newborn's nails are quite delicate and should come off with little problem.

The second part of your baby's body that you may have trouble with is its belly button. I know that you love your baby and think it's the cutest one ever to be born in the history of babies. You revel in every part of its tiny body. Every part that is, except its belly button. I shouldn't even call it a belly button. It's actually that shriveled-up, dried-out, umbilical cord stub that sits on top of the belly button.

Personally, I thought that stub was really gross. I was told to clean it out with alcohol at every diaper change and, in a couple of weeks, it would fall off. But I didn't. I cleaned it out only a couple of times a day, whenever I got the nerve to actually touch the thing. I figured that was good enough.

But as it turned out it wasn't. Soon, my daughter's belly button started to smell. I took her to the doctor and he told me that it was getting infected. He lifted the stubby nub up higher than I had ever lifted it before and I could see the infection setting in. What had I done to my innocent little child?

Luckily, the infection wasn't that bad. The pediatrician told me that if I cleaned it often from then on, it would be just fine. He showed me how to clean it out properly, which I am now going to tell you all about.

Yes, you should clean it at *every* diaper change. But, more important, you must clean it correctly. I never pulled the nub up high enough to get underneath it. I would just swab around the edges and that's what caused the problem. After my hygiene lesson, her nub was so clean you could eat dinner off of it.

After a couple of weeks, it fell off and I didn't have to worry about it anymore. I know this may sound gross, but I saved the stub after it fell off. I keep it in a box where it will one day be joined by a lock of her hair and all of her baby teeth. This way, not only will I have some treasured keepsakes, but I will also have the option of gluing all the stuff together one day if I ever decide I want a second kid. It sounds so much easier than the whole pregnancy and delivery thing.

Sex after the Last Trimester

The best way that I can describe sex after the baby's born is infrequent and painful. For one thing, your sex drive is in neutral. And for another, you're quite sore from having pushed a fruit though your "looms."

Sex isn't even an issue for the first month and a half. After you deliver your baby, your doctor may advise you not to have sex until he sees you in six weeks. It's called the six-week checkup and it can conjure up more stress than cutting your baby's fingernails. During the six-week checkup, your doctor will let you know if you're ready to have sex again.

The visit itself is quick and painless. By the time I went back for my appointment, my regular puffy fingered doctor was back at work after his surgery and feeling fine. He told me how sorry he was for not being there to deliver my baby, and I threatened him with a lawsuit. Not really, but I sure made him feel guilty about it. He took a quick peek inside me and poked around a bit. I think he wanted to make sure the other doctor didn't leave any extra baby parts inside me like a bad mechanic after re-assembling a car.

My doctor told me that things looked good and that I could start having sex again. This surprised me. I was still quite sore, plus things weren't quite lined up down there the way they used to be. I was sure that I'd be given more time to heal before I jumped back on the saddle again (with my panty liners and toilet seat cover, of course). But whether I liked it or not, the doctor said that I was cleared for take-off.

My husband knew that I was going in for my six-week checkup, and he eagerly awaited the news. The poor thing was like a starved dog awaiting a biscuit. I, on the other hand, was like a dog that's had its eyes pinned open for six weeks feeding her puppies around the clock. The last thing I craved was a biscuit. But, against my better judgment, I told my husband the truth about what the doctor said.

As the big event neared, I was reminded of the night that I lost my virginity. In a way, the two evenings were very much alike. Both then and now, I just wanted to get it over with. And both then and now, I knew it was going to hurt.

To prepare myself, I headed down to the local sex-shop for some heavy-duty lubricant. I knew Crisco just wasn't going to do it for me this time. Although I did find what I needed (Astroglide), I also found out that you can't bring an infant into a sex shop. They are quite strict about their rule that you must be over eighteen to enter.

That night I had a glass of wine and things started off quite nicely. But it wasn't long before things came to a crashing halt. Something happened that night that had never happened before in my life. I didn't notice it at first. All I knew was that my husband started to laugh. This is not the reaction I was hoping for especially with my postpartum figure. Insulted, I turned the lights on and noticed that he was covered with breast milk. Yes, it seems that foreplay does indeed get the juices flowing. We both laughed pretty hard because there just wasn't much else we could have done.

After putting on enough nursing pads to absorb Lake Erie, we continued. For him, things got hot and heavy pretty quickly. For me, I was doing my best not to fall asleep. Suddenly, that task got much easier thanks to an incredibly sharp pain. It seems that the lubricant, as heavy duty as it was, wasn't heavy duty enough. We applied more in hopes of making it easier, and although I was as greasy as bad Chinese food, I still felt pain. We thought it best to call it a night and try again in a few days.

The pain that you may experience feels somewhat like an Indian Burn—the politically incorrect name for when someone grabs your forearm with both fists, and twists them in opposite directions. It didn't matter how slowly my husband went in, every little bit hurt. The good news is that once that territory was invaded, it didn't hurt anymore up to that point. It was like getting into a really cold pool. Once you got your toes used to the temperature, then you could put in your entire foot. And so on and so on until you were completely submerged.

The pain of postpartum sex is due in part to your body's decreased estrogen level, made even lower if you're breast-feeding. Less estrogen means a thinner vaginal wall. The amount of pain that you'll experience may also depend upon the kind of delivery that you had. In general, you'll have the least amount of pain during sex if you had a cesarean. You can expect more with a vaginal birth, and even more if an episiotomy, forceps, or a vacuum was needed. I wish I could tell you that the next time we had sex everything went smoothly, but it didn't. It took many times and many weeks, and many tubes of lubricant before we were swimming in the deep end of that pool again.

Sleep Deprivation

Sleep deprivation is by far the worst part about childrearing. I know that you've probably heard how tired new mothers can be, but until it happens to you, these are only hollow words. Of course, it doesn't happen to the same degree for all moms since some newborns sleep more than others. The supposed rule of thumb is that the more the kid weighs, the more hours that he can sleep without needing to be fed. Also, newborns tend to sleep for longer stretches at a time if they drink formula. Breast milk is like milk, but formula is like a milkshake.

My daughter, weighing in at approximately 6½ pounds and breastfed to boot, needed to eat a lot throughout the night—every two hours during the first month. A feeding went something like this:

Midnight. Baby cries. Take her out of the bassinet and into the nursery. Change the dirty diaper and nurse.

12:40 P.M. Baby is taken care of. Attempt to get her back to sleep. If I'm lucky, this takes about ten minutes.

12:50 A.M. Crawl back into my bed and try to put myself back to sleep. This could be quite a feat. You'd think that if a body were tired enough it would fall asleep quickly, but I found the opposite to be true. In the back of my mind, I knew that the baby was going to wake up soon so I had to hurry. It's like having to pee when you're being watched. If there's too much pressure, you just can't perform.

Somewhere around 1:20 A.M. Drift off to sleep.

2:00 A.M. Baby wakes up and wants to be fed again.

This cycle would go on and on throughout the night, every night, month after month. I was so tired that everytime I blinked, my eyes felt as if they were going to bleed.

People would ask me all the time if I could believe that I was a mom. "Don't you just stare at your daughter all day long?" What they don't realize is that if I had any downtime at all, I wouldn't waste it looking at my kid. I would try to get some shut-eye. I know I sound harsh, but it's true. As cute as George Clooney is, I'd resent him too if he demanded to be fed every two hours.

I became jealous of anyone who didn't have a newborn. I started to miss my old life and would fantasize about being a prisoner in solitary confinement. There I'd be, left all alone with no one wanting or needing anything from me. I could get eight hours of continuous shut-eye and wouldn't have to cook or clean. I didn't understand how solitary confinement could be construed as a form of punishment, and began to question the entire judiciary system.

The absolute worst part of sleep deprivation that you'll encounter will be when your baby goes through a growth spurt. This typically happens every three weeks up to, and including, the twelfth week. When the growth spurt struck, my daughter had to be fed *every single hour!* The growth spurt only lasted for a couple of days, but oh, what memorable days they were. I now understand why some people go out for a pack of cigarettes and never come back.

In addition to my crying baby, I was also awakened by my snoring husband. And since I couldn't silence my kid, I had to do something about my husband's face. After much begging, pleading, and threats with sharp objects, my wonderful husband agreed to surgery. Little did he know he'd have to endure two laser surgeries, one radio-wave procedure, and the straightening out of his deviated septum. The good news is that he doesn't snore anymore. The bad news is that he doesn't have much of a face left. But face or no face, I love him anyway and am grateful for all he went through so that I could get a better night's sleep.

The only bit of advice I have to counteract sleep deprivation is one that you've no doubt heard before. Sleep whenever you can. If your baby naps, you nap. I know that this seems obvious, but it can be a difficult thing to do. For even if you're good at falling asleep quickly, you may not want to nap when the house is such a mess. You may think other things are more important than sleeping—like taking a shower, doing laundry, or cooking dinner. But the truth is nothing is more important than recharging your batteries. If you're too tired to function, you're not doing anyone, including your baby, any good.

I was having a really tough time with sleep deprivation after the first couple of weeks. I was a zombie—an engorged, brain-dead, irritable zombie. I didn't see any way to escape from this vicious cycle of sleep deprivation until a wonderful thing happened. My husband caught a really bad cold.

Because of this, he slept in the other room and I kept the baby with me in bed.

We tried before to have our daughter sleep with us. We thought it would be cozy. But although she slept longer, I was the one who suffered. All the while my husband was in slumberland, I was a nervous wreck. For one thing, I was afraid that I'd roll right on top of her. And, if I ever did manage to doze off, she would awaken me with her tiny, yet razor-sharp fingernails. I'd try to scoot over but she'd find me like a heat-seeking missile.

But now with my husband in the other room, there was plenty of bed space for me to sprawl around in. I didn't have the fear of flattening our daughter like roadkill, or getting my body clawed up like I was sleeping next to Freddie Kruger. It was also easier to nurse with her next to me. No need to get out of bed, or transfer her into a bassinet. I would just roll over, stick a breast in her mouth, and fall back to sleep.

But as luck would have it, my husband got better. So it was in with him and out with the baby. If I were to have another child (yeah, right), I would spend the first six weeks with the baby in my bed and the husband out of it. By the end of six weeks, the baby won't be demanding to be fed so often, and the husband will be demanding to return—especially if you've passed your six-week checkup.

Having your baby sleep in bed with you is controversial. Some say that it will wreck your sex life (as if it's not already wrecked). Others say that you'll have lots of problems whenever you move your kid into its own bed. It's a personal decision that only you and your bed partner can make. But even though having a baby in your bed is controversial, the safety precautions are not. All agree that if you have a baby in your bed, you must keep it away from comforters, pillows, and anything else that could obstruct its breathing.

Muscle Soreness

Although I've made no attempt to hide the bitterness I felt toward Mother Nature when I was pregnant, she was beginning to get in my good graces once again. The reason for this change of heart is that after delivery, Mother Nature becomes your very own personal trainer. She helps get your poor, stretched-out body back into shape.

The first way she does this is to give you your own home gym. This new gym is your baby and although it weighs just a few pounds and may drool from time to time, it gets the job done. It took me a while to realize what was happening. At first, I thought that I was coming down with the flu. My whole body ached and every muscle was sore. This went on for several days and I didn't seem to be getting any better. But then, as I was holding my baby girl in one hand and carrying in groceries with the other, I figured it out. I wasn't sick. I was getting back into shape.

I've done my share of exercise in my life. I've walked around the world on the treadmill and climbed to heaven and back on the StairMaster. But never in my life have I been as sore as when I had a newborn. By the end of the day, I had done the equivalent of a major aerobic workout.

I exercised my upper body while hooking bouncy chairs to doorjambs, and my lower body by carrying my baby on my chest while picking up toys from the floor. I must have done 100 squats and 1,000 lunges every day and I wasn't even aware of it! After a few weeks, my thighs were built up enough to lift myself and my kid off the ground without using my hands (you'll find this to be an important maneuver). And in time, my arms became so cut that I could use them to slice deli meat.

If your body feels like you're training for a marathon, there are some things you can do to feel better:

- Take Tylenol.
- Take a hot bath. (Yeah! You can take hot baths again!)
- Use a heating pad.
- Use a product like Ben-Gay to relieve your sore muscles.
- Get a massage.

Another way Mother Nature gets you back in shape is through breastfeeding. She's arranged it so that when your baby nurses, your uterus contracts, enabling it to shrink back

> **"** After I delivered I was still really big for a long time.
> My dad came to visit and he kept poking at my stomach
> and asking if I'm sure there's not another one in there. **"**
> —Nicole

to its original size. If you don't breastfeed, your uterus will still shrink back, but it may take a bit longer.

Keep in mind, this breastfeeding thing is no miracle worker. Even though it may shrink the size of your uterus, it doesn't shrink much else of you. And don't listen to mothers who tell you otherwise. Sure there are those who credit their gigantic postpartum weight loss to breastfeeding, but I think it's due more to genetics than lactation. For plenty of other women like myself, it's the breastfeeding that keeps the weight on.

When I was breastfeeding, I was hungry all the time. Although I tried to diet several times, I could never stick with it. Mother Nature can be cruel, but she's no dummy. She likes her new moms to be a bit plump so they'll have plenty of stored calories to make milk in case her food supply runs out (she made these rules before there were 7-11s on every corner). For me, it wasn't until after I stopped breastfeeding that the weight came off, and, with no dieting required. I'm still not back to my prepregnancy weight, but I'm hopeful.

Reconcilable Differences

There's another thing to prepare yourself for that you may not have been warned about. Sometimes, after having a baby, you and your husband may do a lot of fighting. For although bringing home a baby may make your family feel complete, it may also make your home a very loud place. I know our house was.

❝ We insisted on having dinner out once a week
to keep the romance alive. Once, when the baby-
sitter canceled, we brought our dinner plates, a
candle, and the baby monitor into the back of our
SUV and had a romantic evening in the garage. **❞**
—Lindsey

We fought a lot the first months. What with the major
sleep deprivation, the raging hormones (especially since I
was breastfeeding), and the limited amount of alone time that
we had (basically, while we were sleeping), it's a wonder that
we stayed together.

We fought about a lot of little things that seemed quite
important at the time. We fought about the right way and
wrong way to bathe our child. We fought about how to get
her to stop crying. We fought about who did the most work
and who got the most breaks. There was a constant mental
tally of who did what and when.

Now that things have settled down, I can look back on
those days and realize just how stressful a time it really was. I
was jealous that my husband got to go to work while I had to
stay home with the crying baby. He had lunches; I had dirty
diapers. He had stimulating conversation; I sang "Itsy Bitsy
Spider" 100 times a day. If your home is turning into a battle-
field, there are some things you can do to help quiet things
down:

1. Spend some time away. Not away from each other
but away from your kid. Hire a sitter and have a weekly date
night. Drop the baby off at Grandma's and take in a movie.
It's very important to spend time as a couple, even if it's

for just an hour or two if you're breastfeeding (if you're a good pumper and your baby can take a bottle, you'll have even more time together). You may think it's selfish, but you're actually giving your baby the gift of parents who stay together.

2. Put away the scorecard and agree to disagree. You think that you do more and he thinks that he does. There are no winners in this game and keeping points will only make matters worse. Besides, you and I both know that you do more than your husband does. Women always do.

3. Try to do fun things with your day. Meet a girl-friend for lunch. Put your baby in a carrier and take a hike. Spend a couple of hours walking around a museum. You need to do things that are stimulating. This will provide mental activity for you during the day so you won't be so reliant on your husband to fill the void.

4. Ask yourself if what you're fighting for will still be important in five years. If you're arguing about how to save for college, fine. But if your battle revolves around the proper way to deal with teething pain, let it go.

5. If you're breastfeeding, have your spouse do a nighttime feeding. Get your baby used to taking a bottle with either breast milk or formula. Give up the same feeding time each night (say the 2:00 A.M. one), and after a few days your body will adjust so that your breasts won't feel so engorged. You have no idea how much better you'll get along after you each get more continuous hours of sleep.

How to Deal with a Crying Baby

It was as certain as a pimple on picture day that our baby would have a fit every night. Of course, there were many other times during the day that she would cry, but every evening from about five to seven, she screamed. My husband was sure that there was something wrong with her. He was starting to take it personally since she would always cry when he came home from work. Personally, I knew that she was fine and that it wasn't his taste in neckties that she was objecting to. She had just found her fussy time.

It would drive us up the wall trying to think of ways to get her to stop. We would try everything we could, but nothing seemed to work. But then one day it happened. It was a day that changed our lives forever. As I was getting out of the shower one evening (the time that I usually got around to taking my morning shower), she started to wail. I held her in one hand and turned the hair blower on with the other. And, suddenly, like a bolt of lightning, my baby stopped crying! The instant that the hair blower was turned on, she was turned off. I had stumbled upon an amazing discovery not unlike Newton with the falling apple thing. From that moment on, my life became easier.

I've heard about other ways to help your child stop crying, but none of them worked as well for us as the hair blower. But if the dryer thing doesn't work for you, here are other things to try:

1. **Turn on the vacuum cleaner.** You'll have a quiet baby *and* no dust bunnies.
2. **Take your baby outside.** Sometimes, the temperature change can shake her out of her mood.
3. **Put her in a bouncy chair** on top of the washing machine during the spin cycle. This cycle may have given you pleasure in the past, but never so much as it will now if it makes your baby stop crying.
4. **Play some loud music.**

5. **Put her in a vibrating bouncy seat.** These things are invaluable. My friend Jamie gave me one and I'm now leaving my car to her when I die.

6. **Check out your baby's eyes.** Once, when I couldn't get her to stop crying, I noticed that there was an eyelash in her eye.

7. **Put her in a battery-operated swing.** Some babies find the repetitive rocking very soothing.

8. **Learn how to give your baby a massage.** Baby massage is supposedly quite relaxing for infants and may calm things down. If your baby doesn't like a massage, get one for yourself.

In short, try anything and everything. You may find that one technique works for a week, and then the magic is gone. Just keep trying. You may stumble on your own falling apple.

The Basics

I used to worry incessantly that I was going to kill my baby. Maybe it was because of all those horrible dreams I had when I was pregnant, but I was terrified that I would cause my daughter bodily harm. After cutting off her finger and causing her navel to smell, I was wondering if my fears were going to come true. What ever made me think that I could raise a child?

But every morning I would wake up and realize that she was still here. And every morning, my fears would lessen just a little bit, until now when I hardly worry at all. My husband has now become the neurotic one in the family. He once wanted me to take our daughter to the doctor because she had bad breath.

There are commonsense safety precautions that you can take, as well as a few basic don'ts, but after that, your baby's health is out of your control. Here's a list of don'ts that were given to me by our pediatrician. I'm sure that you'll be given your own list by your doctor, but you can use mine too. You can never be too careful.

1. **Don't** give your child honey. It has spores in it that could cause serious trouble.

2. **Don't** expose your child to the prolonged direct sunlight for the first six months since his skin is too sensitive to wear sunscreen.

3. **Don't** use bubble bath. Use mild baby soap or just warm water. How dirty can a new baby get anyway?

4. **Don't** bring your newborn to a crowded place (supermarket, mall, ball game) for four to six weeks. It doesn't have a good immune system until then and it deserves a fighting chance not to get sick.

5. **Don't** give your baby water. There's plenty of water in breast milk and formula so that you don't have to supplement. The latest reports indicate that even four ounces of water a day can cause harm to your newborn.

6. **Don't** let your baby sleep on its stomach. If it can't sleep on its back, put it on its side. If it has to sleep on its stomach, talk to your pediatrician.

7. **Don't** use baby powder during diaper changes. It travels through the air and your newborn can breathe it in.

8. **Don't** use laundry detergent that's not specifically designed to wash baby clothes (Dreft and Ivory Snow are the most best-known ones out there). And, while we're on the subject, don't use fabric softeners either.

About the Third Month

About the third month, the fog started to lift. I could finally see the light at the end of the tunnel. I could get a few consecutive hours of sleep. My brain cells were starting to regenerate and I could put together a coherent sentence. I would ask my husband to hand me the potholders, instead of the glove-like-thingies-to-take-out-hot-stuff-with.

About the third month, I started getting my life back on track. I could brush my teeth before noon. I had milk in the fridge that hadn't expired. I remembered to call my sister on her birthday (although I still couldn't manage to get her a gift on time).

About the third month, I held up the outfit that my baby wore home from the hospital and wondered how she was ever small enough to fit into it. She took regular naps and ate at regular times. She could stay in one place three times longer without getting bored. I could drive her to the store without crying once the entire way.

About the third month, my baby had a personality. She started to make adorable cooing sounds. I could converse with her in this special language she created. I could tell if she was hungry or bored just by the sound of her cry. She loved her baths and her favorite toy. I could play peek-a-boo with her and hear a subtle hint of laughter.

About the third month, it hit me how deeply I love my little girl. I realized that I'm going to spend the rest of my life trying to shield her from pain, and that there will never again be one moment where I will come first. I know that from now on, I will sacrifice my needs for hers, and do so willingly and without a moment's thought.

About the third month, I would pick up my daughter and, for the first time, she'd put her tiny arms around my neck.

She'd turn her head to see me when I came into the room, and greet me with a smile that would physically warm my heart. I would hold this tiny creature and she'd look up at me with her precious shining eyes. She'd connect with me like no one had ever done before. I would look at my sweet angel who needs me just as much as I need her, and I realized, that maybe, just maybe, I *could* do this again.

Appendix
Resources List

Baby Gear
___

Baby Bargains: Secrets to Saving 20% to 50% on Baby Furniture, Equipment, Clothes, Toys, Maternity Wear and Much, Much More!: 4th Edition by Denise and Alan Fields. Boulder, CO: Windsor Peak Press, 2001.

Baby's First Year
___

● Books

Callie's Tally: An Accounting of Baby's First Year (Or, What My Daughter Owes Me) by Betsy Howie. New York, NY: J. P. Tarcher/Putnam, 2002.

The Everything® Baby's First Food Book: Tasty, Nutritious Meals and Snacks That Even the Pickiest Child Will Love— From Birth to Age 3, by Janet Mason Tarlov. Avon, MA: Adams Media, 2001.

The Everything® Baby's First Year Book: Complete Practical Advice to Get You and Baby Through the First 12 Months, by Tekla S. Nee. Avon, MA: Adams Media, 2002.

The Girlfriends' Guide to Surviving the First Year of Motherhood: Wise and Witty Advice on Everything from Coping with Postpartum Mood Swings to Salvaging Your Sex Life to Fitting into That Favorite Pair of Jeans by Vicki Iovine. New York, NY: Perigee, 1997.

The Happiest Baby on the Block: The New Way to Calm Crying and Help Your Baby Sleep Longer by Karp Harvey, M.D. New York, NY: Bantam, 2002.

Operating Instructions: Journal of My Son's First Year by Anne Lamott. New York, NY: Pantheon, 1993.

Secrets of the Baby Whisperer: How to Calm, Connect, and Communicate with Your Baby by Tracy Hogg with Melinda Blau. New York, NY: Ballantine, 2002.

What to Expect the First Year by Arlene Eisenberg, et. al. New York, NY: Workman Publishing Company, 1989.

Your Child's Health: The Parents' Guide to Symptoms, Emergencies, Common Illnesses, Behavior and School Problems by Barton D. Schmitt, M.D., F.A.A.P. New York, NY: Bantam Books, 1991.

Bed Rest During Pregnancy

● Books

The Pregnancy Bed Rest Book: A Survival Guide for Expectant Mothers and Their Families by Amy E. Tracy. New York, NY: Berkley Books, 2001.

● Organizations

SideLines
P.O. Box 1808
Laguna Beach, CA 92652
949-497-2265
✍*www.sidelines.org*

Birth Defects

● Books

Choosing Naia: A Family's Journey by Mitchell Zuckoff. Boston, MA: Beacon Press, 2002.

Expecting Adam: A True Story of Birth, Rebirth, and Everyday Magic by Martha Beck. New York, NY: Berkley Publishing Group, 2000.

● Organizations

Developmental Delay Resources
4401 East-West Highway, Suite 207
Bethesda, MD 20814
✍*www.devdelay.org*

The National Down Syndrome Society
666 Broadway
New York, NY 10012
212-460-9330
✐*www.ndss.org*

**National Information Center for Children and
Youth with Disabilities**
P.O. Box 1492
Washington, DC 20013
800-695-0285
✐*www.nichcy.org*

Breastfeeding

● **Books**

*The Everything® Breastfeeding Book: Basic Techniques and
Reassuring Advice Every New Mother Needs to Know*
by Suzanne Fredregrill with Ray Fredregrill. Avon, MA:
Adams Media, 2002.

*La Leche League International: The Breastfeeding Answer
Book, 3rd Revised Edition* by Nancy Mohrbacher and Julie
Stock. Schaumburg, IL: La Leche League International, 1997.

So That's What They're For! Breastfeeding Basics by Janet
Tamaro. Avon, MA: Adams Media, 1998.

The Womanly Art of Breastfeeding, 6th Revised Edition by La
Leche League International. New York, NY: Plume, 1997.

• Organizations

La Leche League International
1400 N. Meacham Road
Schaumburg, IL 60173-4808
847-519-7730
✎ *www.lalecheleague.org*

Childbirth

• Books

Baby Catcher: Chronicles of a Modern Midwife by Peggy Vincent. New York, NY: Scribner, 2002.

A Good Birth, A Safe Birth: Choosing and Having the Childbirth Experience You Want by Diana Korte and Roberta Scaer. Boston, MA: Harvard Common Press, 1992.

Pregnancy, Childbirth and the Newborn: The Complete Guide by Penny Simkin, Janet Whalley, and Ann Keppler. New York, NY: Meadowbrook, 2001.

Six Practical Lessons for an Easier Childbirth, 3rd Revised Edition by Elizabeth Bing. Cambridge, MA: Harvard Common Press, 1992.

The Thinking Woman's Guide to a Better Birth by Henci Goer. New York, NY: Perigee Publishing, 1999.

• Organizations

American College of Nurse-Midwives
818 Connecticut Avenue, NW, Suite 900
Washington, DC 20006
888-MIDWIFE
www.midwife.org

The American College of Obstetricians and Gynecologists
409 12th Street, SW
Washington, DC 20024-2188
202-638-5577
www.acog.org

Doulas of North America
P.O. Box 626
Jasper, IN 47547
206-324-5440
www.dona.org

Lamaze International
2025 M Street, Suite 800
Washington, DC 20036
202-857-1128
www.lamaze.org

Midwives Alliance of North America
4805 Lawrenceville Highway
Lilburn, GA 30047
888-923-6262
www.mana.org

National Association of Childbearing Centers
3123 Gottschall Road
Perkiomenville, PA 18074
215-234-8068
215-234-8068
✐*www.birthcenters.org*

Exercise During Pregnancy

● Books

Exercising Through Your Pregnancy by James F. Clapp III.
Omaha, NE: Atticus Books, 2002.

Pregnancy Fitness by the editors of *Fitness* magazine. New
York, NY: Three Rivers Press, 1999.

● Videos

Kathy Smith—Pregnancy Workout
Studio: Sony Wonder
Available in DVD and VHS.

● Web Sites

Fit Pregnancy
✐*www.fitpregnancy.com*

Fertility

● Books

Living with P.C.O.S.: Polycystic Ovary Syndrome by Angela Boss, et al. Omaha, NE: Addicus Books, 2001.

Taking Charge of Your Fertility: The Definitive Guide to Natural Birth Control, Pregnancy Achievement, and Reproductive Health: Revised Edition by Toni Wechsler. New York, NY: Quill, 2002.

● Organizations

American Society for Reproductive Medicine (ASRM)
Formerly the American Fertility Society
1209 Montgomery Hwy.
Birmingham, Al 35216-2809
205-978-5000
✍ *www.asrm.org*

RESOLVE: The National Infertility Association
1310 Broadway
Somerville MA 02144
888-623-0744
✍ *www.resolve.org*

Midlife Pregnancy

● Books

The Complete Guide to Pregnancy after 30: From Conception to Delivery—All You Need to Know to Make the Right Decisions by Carol Winkelman. Avon: Adams Media, 2002.

Miscarriage

● Books

Motherhood after Miscarriage by Dr. Kathleen Diamond.
Avon, MA: Adams Media, 1991.

*Trying Again: A Guide to Pregnancy after Miscarriage,
Stillbirth, and Infant Loss* by Ann Douglas. Dallas, TX: Taylor
Publishing, 2000.

*When a Baby Dies: The Experience of Late Miscarriage,
Stillbirth, and Neonatal Death* by Nancy Kohner. New York,
NY: Routledge, 2001.

● Organizations

SHARE Pregnancy and Infant Loss Support, Inc.
National SHARE Office
St. Joseph Health Center
300 First Capitol Drive
St. Charles, MO 63301-2893
800-821-6819 or 636-947-6164
✍*www.nationalshareoffice.com*

Motherhood

● Books

American Mom: Motherhood, Politics, and Humble Pie by
Mary Kay Blakely. Chapel Hill, NC: Algonquin Books, 1994.

*Life after Birth: What Even Your Friends Won't Tell You
About Motherhood* by Kate Figes. New York, NY: St. Martin's
Press, 2001.

Life's Work: Confessions of an Unbalanced Mom by Lisa
Belkin. New York, NY: Simon & Schuster, 2002.

Multiple Births

• Organizations

The National Organization of Mothers of Twins Clubs
877-540-2200
✍*www.nomotc.org*

The Triplet Connection
P.O. Box 99571
Stockton, CA 95209
209-474-0885
✍*www.tripletconnection.org*

Nutrition During Pregnancy

• Books

*Nutrition and Pregnancy: A Complete Guide from
Preconception to Post-Delivery* by Judith E. Brown. Los
Angeles: Lowell House; Chicago: Contemporary Books, 1997.

Postpartum Depression

• Books

*Depression after Childbirth: How to Recognize, Treat, and
Prevent Postnatal Depression* by Katharina Dalton with Wendy
Holton. New York, NY: Oxford University Press, 2001

Pregnancy

● Books

The Everything® Pregnancy Book, 2nd Edition by Paula Ford-Martin with Elisabeth A. Aron, M.D., F.A.C.O.G. Avon, MA: Adams Media, 2003.

The Girlfriends' Guide to Pregnancy: Or Everything Your Doctor Won't Tell You by Vicki Iovine. New York: Pocket Books, 1995.

What to Expect When You're Expecting: 3rd Edition by Heidi Eisenberg Murkoff, et al. New York: Workman Pub., 2002.

Your Pregnancy Week by Week: 4th Edition by Glade B. Curtis. Tucson, AZ: Fisher Books, 2000.

● Web Sites

iVillage and iVillage chatroom
✍*www.iVillage.com*

ParentsPlace.Com Interactive Pregnancy Calendar
✍*www.parentsplace.com/pregnancy/calendar*

Pregnancy Today: The Journal for Parents-to-Be
✍*www.pregnancytoday.com*

Sexuality

● Books

Dr. Ruth's Pregnancy Guide for Couples: Love, Sex, and Medical Facts by Ruth K. Westheimer. New York, NY: Routledge, 1999.

Single Parenting

• Books

The Complete Single Mother: Reassuring Answers to Your Most Challenging Concerns: 2nd Edition by Andrea Engber and Leah Klungess, Ph.D. Avon, MA: Adams Media, 2000.

Operating Instructions: Journal of My Son's First Year by Anne Lamott. New York, NY: Pantheon, 1993.

• Organizations

The National Organization of Single Mothers
P.O. Box 68
Midland, NC 28107
704-888-KIDS
E-mail: *solomother@aol.com*
✑*www.singlemothers.org*

Parents Without Partners
National. Founded 1957. Membership organization of divorced parents, regardless of the age of the children, and widowed persons.
401 N Michigan Ave.
Chicago, IL 60611
1-800-637-7974
✑*www.parentswithoutpartners.org*

Index